Solution Art

by the same author

Presence and Process in Expressive Arts Work
At the Edge of Wonder
Herbert Eberhart and Sally Atkins
Foreword by Paolo Knill
ISBN 978 1 84905 957 2
eISBN 978 0 85700 811 4

Principles and Practice of Expressive Arts Therapy
Toward a Therapeutic Aesthetics
Paolo Knill, Ellen G. Levine and Stephen K. Levine
ISBN 978 1 84310 039 3
eISBN 978 1 84642 032 0

of related interest

New Developments in Expressive Arts Therapy
The Play of Poiesis
Edited by Ellen G. Levine and Stephen K. Levine
ISBN 978 1 78592 247 3
eISBN 978 1 78450 532 5

SOLUTION ART

A Textbook of Art- and Resource-Oriented Work

Paolo J. Knill
and
Herbert Eberhart

Translated by Wayne Sutherland
Foreword by Margo Fuchs Knill

Jessica Kingsley Publishers
London and Philadelphia

First published in Germany in 2010 by Vandenhoeck & Ruprecht
First published in the English language in Great Britain
in 2023 by Jessica Kingsley Publishers
An imprint of John Murray Press

1

A CIP catalogue record for this title is available from the
British Library and the Library of Congress

ISBN 978 1 83997 760 2
eISBN 978 1 83997 761 9

Printed and bound by CPI Group (UK) Ltd, Croydon, CR0 4YY

Jessica Kingsley Publishers' policy is to use papers that are natural, renewable and recyclable products and made from wood grown in sustainable forests. The logging and manufacturing processes are expected to conform to the environmental regulations of the country of origin.

Jessica Kingsley Publishers
Carmelite House
50 Victoria Embankment
London EC4Y 0DZ

www.jkp.com

John Murray Press
Part of Hodder & Stoughton Limited
An Hachette UK Company

Contents

Foreword by Margo Fuchs Knill 11

Foreword to the original publication by Jürgen Kriz 15

Introduction by the translator 19

1. Introduction 25
   1.1 Where language and artistic-playful activity meet 25
   1.2 Our intended audience 34
   1.3 Background of the authors 35
   1.4 Getting started at different points as well as cross-reading 36
   1.5 And finally thanks to... 37

2. The Idea of Going Together 39
   2.1 Thirty years ago 39
   2.2 The obvious 40
   2.3 Differences 44
   2.4 Where we are today 47
   2.5 The implications for professionals and diverse approaches 48

3. The Extraordinary Experience of (the) World in Counseling and Therapy 55
   3.1 Counseling as a ritual of reconnection—an anthropological view 55
   3.2 Things that are common to all professional counseling 57

3.3 Decentering—a step out of the narrowness of the predicament 61
3.4 Play and the artistic process 63
3.5 General considerations of our practice 69
3.6 Relationship as the foundation 72

4. The Actual Process of a Session 81
4.1 The architecture of the counseling session 81
4.2 Clarification of assignment 89
4.3 The concern and the resources 94
4.4 The vision of a good result 106
4.5 Bridging 117
4.6 Decentering—challenge and motivation 120
4.7 Analysis and feedback in decentering 144
4.8 Yield for the everyday context—the "harvest" 154
4.9 Sustainable continuation 170

5. Fundamental Reflections on Language, Art, and Play 179
5.1 On the use of language 179
5.2 Art and play 186
5.3 Artistic and playful activity in decentering 189
5.4 Talk is silver; action is gold 191

6. Metadiscourse on the Method and Its Effect 193
6.1 Focus of attention 194
6.2 Effects and sustainability 197
6.3 Theoretical thoughts on the effectiveness 205

7. The Application and Its Limits 219
7.1 Areas of application 219
7.2 Limits 233

8. The Origins. 238
8.1 The phenomenological thinking and the development of the art-oriented practice 238

8.2 The art- and expressiveness-oriented practice and the critique of other methods contained therein 251
8.3 The Focus on Solutions practice and its tradition of thought 254
8.4 Focus on Solutions and its criticism of other methods 273

9. Professional Requirements and Considerations on Continuing Education and Professional Development. . . . 277
9.1 Requirements for the counselor 277
9.2 Thoughts on continuing education and professional development 280

10. The Seriousness of Play and the Surprise of Art—Concluding Thoughts. 288

References 292

Index. 297

Foreword by Margo Fuchs Knill

Yes
must be more than an option.

Let's get up, every day
and hold the Yes
in front of us
a shield of kindness
I am here with you,
my sister, my brother
my global family.

Let's get up, every day
walk through the fields
without kicking the grass.

Let's give each other
another chance
and act differently
replace the "must" with "we can."

How else could we look spring
gracefully into her blossoming eyes?

Margo Fuchs Knill

Let's face it—we are challenged worldwide by a pandemic crisis, still. What used to work doesn't work anymore, and the new direction is up in the air. Fear and uncertainty are spreading due to economic and social disruptions. Job loss, poverty, and mental health issues are on the rise: from depression to insomnia to increased levels of alcohol and drug use to violence in families. On the other side, times of heightened challenge are also periods of heightened creativity, innovation, and modernization. In *Solution Art (Lösungskunst)*, Paolo Knill and Herbert Eberhart present how their art- and rhetoric-based methodology enables struggling people to have a voice. Knill and Eberhart's professional coaching, consulting, and supervisory work, based on a theory of practice, empowers clients to have a say in their own development and build their capacity to generate new solutions.

We can proudly say that the field of expressive arts is established globally, in theory and in practice. To date, many schools and practitioners are well trained in applying the arts within mental health practices and institutions, international communities and organizations, conflict transformation and peacebuilding initiatives, sustainable development, and climate action movements.

The content—the arts—is crucial; however, maybe even more so is the professional change agent's ability to be skillful and efficient in communicating what s/he is going to do and why. Knill and Eberhart emphasize that this takes more than being expressive and passionate about creating with the arts. Professionals have an ethical and esthetical responsibility towards their clients, their artistic process, and their product. Without a depth of understanding about this responsibility, expressive arts practitioners risk, albeit unintentionally, causing harm to those they aim to help. A phenomenological and resource-oriented analysis allows a multisensory approach to meaning-making rather than reducing the artwork to a "problem-tranced" reflection. This demands nonjudgmental, inclusive language when facilitating a session, a rhetoric that invites new perspectives and validates the diversity and uniqueness of each individual, team, or community seeking help.

This book is about both the verbal *and* nonverbal levels of expressive arts, for they are intertwined. Language is power; artistic expression is power. Moving forward, the only chance we have to successfully address personal, communal, organizational, institutional, and global crises is to evolve how we communicate about them; how we communicate *through* them. The authors serve as role models, presenting readers with experiential wisdom about how to approach the development of lingual skills *while* working with the arts. They use language in an explorative, enriching, even orally traditional way, yet with scientific precision. Their style helps to avoid theoretical jargon as well as lengthy, over-simplified lists of dos and don'ts.

Even though an expressive arts professional focuses on works of art and the process of creating, there is no way around language. Language matters—even more so when you tap into nonverbal realms. Professionals cannot avoid cultivating clear, clean, and supportive language when facilitating sessions. Doing so is vital in protecting the emerging work of art from what Shaun McNiff calls "image abuse." Even though the expressive arts methodology is different from a "talking cure," it, too, takes well-educated verbal skills to make a session effective. Knill and Eberhart thus introduce the notion of "linguistic enrichment." They show how change agents can refrain from platitudes and generalizations by employing an explicit, differentiated, rich language that also strengthens esthetic, sensorial resonance. The different use of language creates a different reality for the client, a reality nourished by life quality.

I must admit, I have been skeptical about whether a translation of *Lösungskunst* could relay the dense and lively content of the book. I am grateful for the way in which this translation allows the original content to shine forth, fundamentally capturing both the novelty of thought and the beautiful simplicity of the argument. The translator, Wayne Sutherland, masterfully carves out the different rhetoric styles. *Solution Art* is more than a translation of something previously written; it is a new *oeuvre*, an artwork in and of itself, because it captures the dynamic, dialogical spirit of the authors.

Solution Art is an inspiring hands-on textbook that offers a thorough foundation for further research. The book is not only *about* a solution-based language and resource-oriented use of expressive arts; it *embodies* a theory of practice by sharing lived examples of dialogue, discourse, case study, and lecture style. The reader is even welcomed to "attend" a passionate, interdisciplinary symposium facilitated by Knill and Eberhart. They show the professional and the layperson alike methods for activating potential and gaining new insights. Their concept of *decentering* is precise yet able to describe more than just technique, grounding in arts-based mindfulness the notion of *the third*, and artistic co-creation.

It is precisely the hybrid linguistic style of this textbook that propels a forward-thinking urgency. *Solution Art* speaks to the academically interested person as well as to the practitioner who wants to see it work in practice. It connects with anyone who loves to excavate the expressive arts' field's multiple foundations, critically reflect on its philosophical underpinnings, and advance the work further. *Solution Art* satiates the reader who seeks a shortcut to understanding the definitions of expressive arts' key terminology.

Humans have always turned to something else, a third force, when they find themselves at a dead end. Knill and Eberhart unlock creative thinking. They emphasize that understanding the question itself already gives answers. I am convinced that our contemporary world—especially as we learn from the Covid pandemic crisis—needs this kind of thoughtful balance between encouraging innovative advancement and establishing a well-considered theory of practice. This open-ended textbook helps the relatively new field of expressive arts to stay fresh and exciting.

Paolo Knill is known for his strong ability to "break circles," let go of what is no longer working, and let the new in—"to not calcify," as he would say. Herbert Eberhart is known for his endlessly youthful curiosity, for never being satisfied with an easy answer, for always seeking the deeper, truer questions. *Solution Art* is about more than "searching and finding solutions." In this book, we learn about methods that allow sustainable change by letting go of seeking it.

Schaffhausen, December 2021

Foreword to the original publication by Jürgen Kriz

We live in a time that demands con-centration from people—perhaps as a countermovement to increasing globalization, internationalization, information overload, and bureaucratic hyper-complexity. This often means that the manifold stimuli are blanked out and are not supposed to distract from the actual task. Quality is to be optimized and thus controlled based on a few measurable parameters. And this is not only in the manufacture of industrial products but also in medical care, psychotherapy, teaching, or a variety of other services. Above all, however, one has to focus more and more on economic efficiency. What happens must be "profitable" and "cost-effective." And what does not "pay off" appears to be superfluous, if not a hindrance.

No doubt, wherever such optimization succeeds, the "business machine" does indeed run faster, the days spent in hospitals during operations are reduced, more counseling sessions can be conducted per day, and more "empirically validated" psychotherapies can be billed per therapist. Many work processes can be simplified and accelerated if one concentrates on the "essentials"—namely, if one leaves out everything "unnecessary" and does not "daydream."

However, such optimization obviously does not always succeed, or it works only for a limited period of time. Particularly when the underlying conditions for the optimized processes and solutions change significantly, the probability of problems or even a collapse of the previously successful approach increases. This is because it must now be determined whether and how the processes that have been so well established can adapt to the new conditions. Since every system—the individual with his or her processes of perception, processing, and action, couples and families with their interaction dynamics, or larger units with their organizational processes—is subject to certain developments, such breaks in the continuity of previous solutions are unavoidable. One can speak of typical "developmental tasks" for the system.

For example, an interaction dynamic between parents and their three-year-old child, however optimal it may be, has to cope with several developmental tasks in the following twenty years (including school enrollment, puberty, adolescence), consisting of a qualitative restructuring of the processes that have functioned well up to now. Clinging to the "tried and true"—if the now 23-year-old is still treated like a three-year-old or even allows himself to be treated like one—obviously presents a substantial problem. Furthermore, an even more "efficient" use of previous process patterns and solution strategies would tend to increase the problem.

In all such cases of reorientation to changed conditions, what is needed is not concentering on previous ways of seeing and doing, but de-centering from their fascinating (or, in systemic jargon, attracting) influence. A hundred years ago, for example, Gestalt psychologists showed that creative and productive thinking requires stepping back and letting go of constricting, ingrained ways of looking at things, which is why creative ideas and solutions not infrequently come up in the shower or while falling asleep. Such "aha" experiences presuppose the dissolution of previous views and problem-solving structures—that is, greater complexity and uncertainty—so that something can be rearranged. Seemingly unnecessary things and "daydreaming in this direction" now become important moments that promote adaptive reorientation.

If we now consider how many systems and system levels a person is involved in (perceiver, thinker, feeler, doer, interactor as partner, mother, secretary, club chairman, etc.), and take into account that all these systems are confronted with new developmental tasks from time to time, we can only marvel at how well the inevitable changes function in our world. We, as therapists, consultants, and coaches, are only contacted by those "systems" where the adaptation to new conditions does not work, or the development tasks are not solved adequately.

However, the social trend toward concentration in the service of efficiency, which is often only superficially oriented, described above—perhaps too pointedly—is not exactly a good breeding ground for the promotion and development of the decenterings that are so important. The principles and metaphors in the economically dominated discourses of our living environment are interspersed with the terms placed in quotation marks above, which for their part act as sense attractors and hardly help to expand the spaces of understanding and solutions but rather narrow them. People then behave all too much like the cartoon of two managers running away in panic from an approaching train on the railroad tracks, shouting to each other, "If a rail switch doesn't come soon, we're doomed!" Instead of just moving faster and faster on well-worn tracks, or presumably hoping in vain for standard alternatives already built in, such as a rail switch, the two would simply have to stop now, decenter, and look at the space to the left and right of the tracks, where there are many new paths. However, the linguistic descriptions of the problem and its solutions—for instance, "How can we run away from the train even faster?"—often obscure the view of unconventional possibilities. Language, with its concepts and structures, contributes to this. For decades, sociologists have been working out how strongly concepts conveyed in language reify and reduce life's vital and complex processes.

This book on the principles and practices of decentering, including intermodal artistic processes, is, therefore, an invaluable contribution to the discourse on how people with "problems" (in the broadest sense) can make use of, or first come into contact with, their resources that have been lost from view. The two authors have decades of practical and teaching experience with the models and approaches developed in this book. In fruitful cooperation, they combine psychological and artistic expertise, each with a different focus. The message is sympathetic to the fact that artistic- and psychological-counseling activities—and even more so the bodies of knowledge to which both perspectives refer in each case—cannot be seamlessly transferred into one another or even easily integrated. There remains a tension—but it can be used fruitfully.

This book also succeeds very well in linking practical, real-life situations, their theoretical elaboration, and the resulting procedures with practice-oriented hints and instructions for action, and the underlying epistemological and methodological roots—in short, a rare and satisfyingly successful interweaving of practical and reflexive or theoretical aspects, considerations, and discourses. These range from the actual process of a session to reflections on language, art and play, the explanatory models for the effect of decentering, and the discussion of the particular context of a counseling situation set up in this way. However, the limits of applicability are also discussed. Furthermore, a separate chapter is also devoted to the question of teaching appropriate skills. Here, it is a question of how art-based decentering processes can be professionally guided or accompanied. Thus, the book is a valuable source for further development and reflection for teachers as well as learners, and for theorists as well as practitioners.

I wish this book well-deserved success. It can give people in many different contexts—whether as teachers or learners, as counselors, therapists or coaches, or simply to stimulate self-support—important hints and encouragement to face life's myriad challenges of growth and development creatively.

Osnabrück (Germany) 2009

Translated by Wayne Sutherland

Introduction by the translator

Translating spoken and written language is not easy.

In recent years, several attempts have been made to translate the book *Lösungskunst* into English. The attempts did not fail because of the 'untranslatability' Walter Benjamin referred to in his essay "The task of the translator."[1]

The translation attempts failed because of the somewhat unclear premise of what this translation should achieve.

During my work, I came to the conclusion that it is not necessary to rewrite *Lösungskunst*, to elevate it quasi-poetically. A simple interpretation is sufficient.

It is a text in the form of a lecture. The text invites the reader to attend, taking notes and asking questions, as they would in a lecture hall. The translator's only requirement is to allow the authors to speak. In this sense, we can follow the demand of Walter Benjamin: that the meaning and the meant are closest when transmitted, as opposed to translated. (Baudelaire, 1923).

It was unnecessary to make an " ideal and definitive 'translation within the expressive arts theoretical framework. Every creative activity, and translation is thereby creative in two ways: on the one hand, the choice of words is a creative decision; on the other hand, the act of translation creates something new. Ultimately, it is not necessary to translate unambiguously; what emerges speaks about itself and of itself. Octavio Paz encourages us to trust the act of translation itself because it is familiar to us.

1 Walter Benjamin, *The Task of the Translator, Selected Writing, Volume 1 1913–1926*, edited by Marcus Bullock and Michael W. Jennings.

"No text can be completely original because language itself, in its very essence, is already a translation: first from the nonverbal world and then because each sign and each phrase is a translation of another sign, another phrase" (Schulte & Biguenet, 1992).

We can only understand "the third," a term coined by the authors of the book 'Lösungkunst'. "The third" is a terminus technicus of this method. It does not matter whether it is a piece of wood, a poem, a dance gesture, or the sound of an oboe. It may sound almost esoteric when we say, "it does something to us—it comes to us—it touches us." A blind person can touch a painting. The faint smell of turpentine on a Tintoretto is as much a part of the work of art as the depiction of the Crucified Christ.

To translate a book is to be *there* and, in that sense, first to leave the authors alone (Schleiermacher, 1838, pp. 207–245). The authors have done their work. We do not need to introduce the reader of this book to the subject. Over the last 30 years, expressive art therapy has become an established and integral part of counseling methods. What we can do with this translation is to invite the reader in. We can give them a direct window into the beginnings of theory and the immediacy of practice. There is something urgent, something crude, almost unfinished about the book *Solution Art*. That's a good thing.

It is a book with the power that only explorers exude. It is often sketchy, quickly noted. And it is not meant to be an endpoint. Rather, its fragmentary style makes it raw material for further research and the reader's experiments. It is a book that conveys the feeling of having broken through a wall. Rubble lies there—and, at the same time, the opening reveals a view of a new world.

The raw material, however, is not arbitrary. The mixture and approach of language and artistic activity as proposed and practiced by the two authors is highly precise in its processes. Unpredictable results indeed emerge. These are the purpose and goal of the method. The architecture of the processes in the design of the therapeutic process is rigid. Only through the narrow framework, the restriction (Gronau & Lagaay, 2010, p. 30), can the liberating impulse be stimulated. The restriction, which as a *Notenge* limits the client, renders him helpless, and becomes in its mirror inversion the entrance to the self-support forces and resources that were invisible and fallow before the artistic interaction.

The therapeutic work, and more comprehensively, the accompanying work with the client, begins in the center of his concern. The support starts at the point where thoughts are circling; feelings cannot find a suitable way out, are tediously repeating themselves, thus reinforcing helplessness. To find a way out, a solution, it is crucial to be able to leave this center. Only on the outside can a new view emerge (Margo Fuchs, 1994). And only by experiencing another possibility of the world, can the potential for shaping the everyday world be perceived.

In this context, the two authors, Herbert Eberhart and Paolo Knill, following Merleau-Ponty (2001), speak of a kind of alternative experience of the world reflected in artistic action through the imagination (Eberhart & Knill, 2010, p. 29).

When we speak of leaving the two authors as undisturbed as possible in translation, this inevitably raises the question of the authors and their language. Without going into biographical details, two authors meet here who complement each other congenially from their different academic backgrounds: Herbert Eberhart, an experienced therapist, social worker, and clinical psychologist, and Paolo Knill, entrepreneur, musician, and natural scientist.

Both meet—as can be read at the beginning of the book—by chance.

Their common question is that of an effective approach to help the client, an approach with a demonstrable and repeatable effect, an approach that can make the client the designer of his own solution. Both authors also have in common that they like to nudge their counterparts with unexpected questions into thinking and doing.

Today, the term "resource-oriented" has become an integral part of modern therapeutic approaches. In the book's writing , if one may put it that way, one can feel the paradigm-shifting postulate of transferring the creative power to the client.

The two authors are Swiss. They write German with Swiss influences and idioms (Helvetism). German often uses passive sentence forms. In translation, these are mostly preserved. The author's intent is conveyed through the use of passive sentence structures, suggesting that they are willing to allow and affirm attitude towards the client and his or her path.

Again, in the translation, I have tried to keep what is meant and the way it is delivered as close as possible to the authors and their idiosyncrasies.

The book "Principles and Practice of Expressive Arts Therapy: Towards a Therapeutic Aesthetics" (2004), published by Jessica Kingsley Publishers, can be considered as a reference to the book *Solution Art*.

This book is a reference text in that it is the first time that long-time faculty members of the European Graduate School, Stephen Levine and Ellen Levine, in collaboration with Paolo Knill, made the main aspects of expressive arts theory available to the English public in book form.

However, it should be noted that Paolo Knill's text has been translated into English in discussion and dialogue. The terms used are explanations and clarifications rather than direct translations. The term *Notenge* can be taken as an example. In "*Principles and Practice of Expressive Arts Therapy*, the term is conveyed as "the helpless situation." The English language has an appropriate term for this distress, that constricts and narrows one's throat: anguish—or, if one wants to expand it—the anguish of worry or concern. The term is etymologically derived from the German *eng* (Pfeifer, 2010).

In the present translation, the core terms of Paolo Knill from *Principles and Practice of Expressive Arts Therapy* have been adopted for the most part. However, these have been taken where obviously better, more accurate, or simply correct alternatives were available. The coherence of the terms is largely preserved. This also intends to introduce the readers and students, who have made their first steps into the theory of expressive arts therapy with the chronologically earlier book in English, to the thematically earlier work *Solution Art* in as undistorted a manner as possible.

In the introduction to *Lösungskunst*, Jürgen Kriz notes how important it is to be able to pause and step out of the current question.

The year 2022 has shown us all that new ways and solutions are needed.

Solutions and new ways can be found in artistic activity and in art-based research. The year 2022 has taken away the words for many things and brought us into a *Notenge*. The fact that this book can now be made available to an English-speaking audience seems particularly important to us.

In the fall of 2020, Paolo Knill passed away.

Paolo Knill was my Ph.D. advisor.

Like Herbert Eberhart and Paolo Knill, we also had different professional and academic backgrounds. Paolo Knill—as mentioned—music, natural sciences, and research in therapy. Myself, social anthropology, communication sciences, psychiatric nursing, and adult education. Together we had experience in the private sector as entrepreneurs. And we also met by chance.

But something that connected us beyond that was fencing. Both Paolo Knill and I—albeit at different times—actively pursued the sport of fencing. It is difficult to convey what fencing is if you have never done it yourself. From the spectator's perspective, it looks elegant and supple. From the inside, it is lightning fast, without hesitation, and powerful.

And fencing is also dangerous. In fact, you meet another person with a weapon and go at him (and—rarely though—there is serious injury—or even death).

The processes of play and interplay with the opponent are important. The challenge, the provocation, the feint.

Because this playfulness is something serious in the truest sense of the word, you always respect the opponent. You have respect for skill, you have respect for danger, and you have respect for people.

Anyone who has observed fencing comrades knows how friendly and straightforward they are with each other. Anything can happen on the fencing piste—when the epee is lowered, it is a rare friendship indeed.

Paolo Knill challenged me often and with pleasure. Some of his brilliant ideas touched me; others I could parry with wit.

We took our game seriously, experiencing the joy and camaraderie that can only come when one recognizes the power of being serious and showing respect for one another.

Paolo Knill and I had lively battles. I insisted that the problem must be fully understood in order to solve it. At the very least, one had to find out whether one wanted to solve the right problem in the first place. With his resource-oriented, decentering approach, Paolo Knill always thought that you had to grasp the problem but step beyond it if you wanted to create or expand the space for solutions.

We never agreed—but we both won.

Translating a seminal work is always a challenge—I think Paolo Knill and I would have agreed on that.

Wayne Sutherland September 2022

1

Introduction

1.1 Where language and artistic-playful activity meet

What happens when the world of the arts and the world of psychology meet, and neither is made subservient to the other? This book results from such a meeting and the outcome of a collaboration that has now lasted more than three decades. The resulting working method is one in which productive synergies are developed through the mindful use of language and through artistic activity. Within counseling and therapy processes, surprising turns can often be observed that open up new perspectives and lead to positive effects.

Psychologists move in language

As psychologists, we move first and foremost in language. We listen to what the other person conveys to us through language, and we try to create an effect through speaking. And even if we are aware that we, as speakers, move on a kind of map and that this map can by no means be equated with the "landscape," the concrete of experience and of experiencing (e.g., Simon, 1991), our understanding and our actions are nevertheless strongly guided by the order of language.

The organizing function of language (e.g., Kriz, 2004) facilitates people's everyday lives enormously. The process of routinely using expressions and sayings enables us to orient ourselves to one another quickly. The fact that we often exchange some kind of language template in the process does not bother us, and we do not notice it in most situations.

The situation is different in counseling and therapy scenarios. When describing areas of concern (see Section 4.3), but especially when describing "good futures" (Section 4.4), an accumulation of stereotypical phrases is noticeable.

Fixed language "scripts" shrink the diversity of perceptions and experiences (language as a dead end)

Language templates, which can also be called "fixed scripts," are usually counterproductive in a counseling situation. In our own words, we speak of a "poor" language (following White, 1989) and strive to guide our clients to a "rich" language.

Those who seek counseling or therapy want to effect change. This usually involves situations characterized by clinging to outdated ways of responding or ways of responding that are not appropriate to the situation. Therefore, what is needed is flexibility or, in the terminology we use, "widening of the scope or play range." A person who is able to report richly in content pays attention to the richness of his world of experience and also pays attention to small differences that can be used, for example, for new things. He is also prepared to elaborate upon ideas and visions and thus make them more accessible to realization.

> For T.T., difficulties, distress, and many limitations are gathered around the word "can." This verb, which triggers positive thoughts and memories in most people, has an extremely ambivalent effect on him and triggers irritation, doubt, and, not infrequently, even fear. This young adult, who apparently had it drilled into him at home that he, unlike his sister, "can't do anything," is suspicious of every sentence that deals with his current ability. He suspects hypocrisy or naive credulity in the praise of a colleague at work, and he hears superficiality or ignorance in a neutral statement by a counselor about his skills. And if he cannot avoid the fact that he has already repeatedly succeeded in something, that he obviously "can" do it, then he fears self-deception and a later rude awakening with corresponding disappointments. There were times in T.T.'s life when even a neutral remark not referring to him personally, in which the word "can" appeared, could cause irritation.

In the everyday language of every person, some expressions or sentences have a large halo of meanings around them and can tie up the attention of the person in question to a substantial degree. This has a negative effect, as in the above example, but can also trigger strong future-oriented forces in a positive sense.

Enrichment through asking concretizing questions

This situation can be addressed by using the skills of professional dialogue. Based on a relationship characterized by "appreciative curiosity," all questions are helpful if they prompt the client to describe details and thereby discover differences in what is supposedly always the same. "Always the same dead ends" that someone reports, for example, then turn out to be always slightly different situations, and it becomes possible to discover an aspect of taking action in one or the other that has had a positive effect and could in principle also be used in other contexts.

The same applies, for example, in coaching to formulate what one to be a good result from the session or the "good future" that one is aiming for. Our clients often have little to say about this—except that the problem will be solved and perhaps a general, vague statement that it will then be "easier." Here, too, concretizing questions and, above all, a simple, repeatedly asked "What else?" help to formulate the imagined positive future more concretely and in more detail. Only then can it really unfold its motivational effects for a transformation in a positive direction.

Artistic activity opens up new dimensions of possibilities

The situation is different and new when artistic activity comes into play. We use this to refer to short, episodic activities, such as a rhythm improvisation with different takes or an installation with everyday objects, in which aesthetic considerations guide the placement of the individual parts.

The way we use artistic elements, with the simplest means and at the same time great presence, accompanied by curious appreciation, results in a process with unusual and surprising turns. At the same time, this process oriented towards what we call "work" primarily makes stereotyped behaviour impossible. The way in which such an activity is introduced and the professional's choice of words (see Section 4.6) stimulate curiosity and experimentation. Reducing so-called essentials is not the goal, but rather enrichment, diversity, and richness of perspective.

If artistic activity is used as an episodic part of a counseling or therapy sequence and is included in the overall process in a certain way, we call this de-centering. This term stands for a temporary distancing from the central concern (de-centering) and—in the procedure described here—turning to an artistic-playful activity. The procedure has been registered as Intermodal Decentering IDEC®. The adjective "intermodal" indicates that different artistic media are used and that something can be enriched and deepened through several disciplines. For example, it is possible to start with a simple piece of sculptural installation, which is then interpreted poetically and finally translated into a movement.

Such a specific, resource-oriented use of art and play in an independent sequence of specific methodological parts opens up surprising perspectives that encourage the client to take lasting steps towards change.

> Norman and Christian form the management team of a private educational institute. Norman is the business manager. Christian oversees curriculum and course planning and is dedicated to research. Both are also active as lecturers and supervisors. They ask the consultant for a half-day counseling session because a "simmering conflict was coming to a head."
>
> In conversation, Norman describes himself as overworked and under pressure, "because the financial resources are simply not enough." Christian "means well," has "a thousand good ideas," but does not understand that these are useless within the situation. Christian does not understand why Norman "hesitates" and "slows down" so much. He is fully committed but does not want to "play the fantasist" in the team.
>
> In response to questions from the counselor, they report that they work well together in some areas. As examples, they mention the new spatial arrangement of the institute or rare situations where they teach together. Asked about the reasons, they say, "We both have the same thing in mind and work methodically in the same way, even if we have different styles." As a good outcome, they would like to be able to decide at the end of the session whether they should continue together as a leadership team. If yes, what should be changed in the collaboration? If no, what kind of managerial organization should be presented to the supervisory board?
>
> The counselor's suggestion to do a music improvisation during

the decentering phase is immediately met with approval. Both have good access to music privately, and musical instruments are available in the room.

Norman chooses the piano as his musical instrument, and Christian chooses the xylophone and his voice. The counselor asks Norman if he would also like to add his voice, but he declines. "Not for the time being," he says.

To explore the instrument and raise awareness, the counselor asks them both to find a short sequence of notes that somehow fascinates them with its arc of tension. He invites them to experiment until a satisfying motif "arrives." This phase concludes with both playing the motif to each other. The sequence of notes composed by Norman is called Motif A, the one composed by Christian Motif B.

Improvisation and Take I: The two motives answer each other hesitantly. The whole begins to flow a bit when Christian uses his voice. He does this by holding the same tone again and again for a longer time (central tone as a connecting element).

The short interim evaluation shows that both experience the "interweaving" of the two motifs as a challenge. The central tone is a help in this. Norman's suggestion to start with both motifs at the same time is accepted.

Improvisation and Take II: The motifs now often sound simultaneously but remain somewhat "stiff." Rhythm and dissonances seem to cause some trouble. The music gains modulation as soon as Norman also uses his voice for the first time.

Intermediate evaluation: Both are dissatisfied with the beginning. On the other hand, they would like to "make music" more with the voice and use the instruments only "as timbre accompaniment."

Two more takes with in-between evaluations follow. Before the last, the fifth take, Norman wants to practice so that his "sound strokes" (fifths and fourths as open chords) leave enough room for Christian's Motif B.

Improvisation and Take V: A surprising dynamic emerges with a continuous pulse that remains alive and organizes a polyphony that is not clearly fixed in tonality and then clearly ends in an open octave.

Now everyone involved finds that "it clicks." They immediately want to improvise again in this way so that the piece can be recorded on tape.

The subsequent aesthetic analysis (Section 4.7) yields a rich description, especially in the analysis of process. In the harvesting phase (Section 4.8), Norman spontaneously says, "Yes, if our leadership team is to function, they should actually both be able to lead from their own motifs in a structure that is clearly developing for both of them." And Christian adds, "And when someone takes the lead, it is helpful if they still give the other person some room to maneuver."

In the final discussion phase, both agree to continue as a team. Specifically, the job specifications are to be revised in terms of responsibility and decision-making authority, and Christian is to receive mentoring from Norman in accounting and budgeting.

L.K. has been working in a good position in the healthcare sector for many years. She is in the second part of a multi-year, in-service training program that will take her out of her traditional career field. She comes to the coaching session quite unsure of what a first step into the new field might look like. As a good outcome of the session, she formulates that she wants to have a "feeling" of what such a step might look like. L.K. is immediately ready to interrupt the conversation and do something "completely different."

The counselor hands her a large sheet of relatively thick, white drawing paper and gives her six minutes to "make something" with it or out of it. She is free to take a second object (e.g., a pair of scissors) from an open rack with all kinds of materials and figures and use it in some way. L.K. is perplexed at first, but then she folds the sheet several times and tries to tear a hole in it. This fails even after several attempts. The paper is too thick. On impulse, L.K. crumples the paper and stamps her feet on it. The material has become "tearable" through this procedure, and an upright sculpture-like structure with a large opening is created. L.K. declares the task finished before the time available to her has expired. The counselor asks her if the work "still needs something." She says no.

Now the counselor asks L.K. to choose a location for herself and her work where the sculpture shows itself "in the best perspective" for the viewer. From this place, she should write down adjectives that come to mind when she sees the sculpture. Following this, she is given time to write a short story including these adjectives.

As a conclusion, L.K. has to choose a new "appropriate place" for herself and the sculpture in the room for the second time, from which she can read the story to an "audience" (here, the counselor).[1]

Further elaboration (see Sections 4.7 and 4.8) leads to a whole series of different associations, from which L.K. selects the item "this animalism in doing" as the most attractive at the time.

In the final conversation, L.K. resolved to deal with her patients differently and "not to be so cautious anymore." She wants to start painting again, do weight training again, and "do something crazy once in a while." Asked about the "feeling for the step to be taken" that she strives for as a "good result," she thinks she has noticed that it somehow has to do with "being allowed to be rough." (L.K. seems graceful in her appearance.)

A telephone inquiry one year later reveals that L.K. has found her way.

Attractive and low-threshold

Artistic non-professionals—which almost all of our clients are—move in artistic-playful activities on a terrain where curiosity and the desire to experiment can still be found. Since no trained artistic or craft skills are required, the threshold for creative experimentation is set low. The professional takes care that the client can fully engage in this different activity and that the whole process leads to a rewarding result.

Thanks to the simplicity of the task, this artistic and playful activity requires neither previous experience in the use of materials and resources nor a high level of skill. Nevertheless, it should be attractive, stimulating, and immediately inviting to action. There must be nothing casual about it.

Art is sense activity

It is the physical-sensory qualities that are in the foreground for us in artistic activity. It is not everyday logic that guides the activities, but

1 Due to the time available, in this case, the "work-like" processing of one of the elements created was waived.

rather sensory stimulation, imagination, surprises, and the joy of being able to surrender to the process, at least temporarily. This process is primarily work-oriented and is determined by what is in the process of being created. Thus, in improvised dance, one step influences the next; in painting, one brushstroke influences the next. However, the process can also be spontaneous and playful—like the actions of a child who, in all seriousness, "lets art emerge" for a few minutes. The satisfaction experienced usually lies in the doing itself, and is less determined by the result.

The immediate effects of the decentering episodes on clients are readily observable, and various senses are addressed. In their actions, they appear very focused, often visibly challenged, but at the same time animated and relaxed, as evidenced by flushed cheeks and sometimes half-suppressed exclamations of amazement.

Art-oriented action understood in this way can also be used with success elsewhere—for example, in the attunement phase of a team session or as an experiment or task to explore and deepen a theme between two sessions.

Art and language enrich each other

With immersion in art and play, people experience reality in a new and different way. In this book, we speak of the "alternative experience of the world" (Section 3.2). Artistic action is guided by a different kind of logic, a logic that emerges through action rather than through reflection before action. Contexts are discovered from within the design process.

It is also central that the "attracting, stabilizing, and reifying meanings of everyday world language" (Kriz, 2007, p.26) are eliminated.

> Ms. G., a 55-year-old music teacher, who has had various therapies over many years and is once again "attempting brief therapy" because of unchanged symptomatology, sees herself as "bad" and as a "failure." After the second session, she is given the task of choosing two or three passages of music that contain something of what she wants to make of her life. She is free to play these passages herself (from sheet music or as improvisations) or to select them from recordings. For the next session, Ms. G. brings a musical example by Rossini and one by Beethoven on two CDs. She reports that she felt happier "than she has

in a long time" when selecting the appropriate CD or the requested passages in the music store. Over and over, she says, it went through her mind: "This is my life." Melodies and rhythms seem to have swept away all self-criticism.

Subsequently, the client processes these musical passages like artistic works that were created during a decentering phase (see Sections 4.7 and 4.8.). The central aspect that emerges from this processing for Ms. G. revolves around the "urge for freedom." This concept becomes both a starting point and a goal orientation for the further successful therapeutic work.

The methodical approach

Ms. G., analogously to her professional activity, engaged with classical art in the pursuit of the assignment, and she did so in a receptive manner. She could also have improvised on her instrument and brought these improvisations with her on a recording. Receptive engagement with given works of art is a possible but rare exception for our approach. We focus on active artistic action, emphasizing the imaginative elements during the decentering phase of a counseling or therapy sequence. In accordance with the usually short time available and the client's previous experiences in the respective medium used, the resulting work does not have to meet any particular artistic criteria. However, it should be appealing.

Taken on its own, artistic work can have a nurturing and healing effect. If this artistic activity is to be used for steps of change, which can be stimulated in counseling and realized in everyday life, an appropriate language is needed. It is an appreciative, resource-oriented, searching language, which—as far as the decentering act and the resulting work are concerned—is oriented towards the terminology of the corresponding creative medium. It is also a language that time and again also takes up formulations and metaphors that were spontaneously used by the clients themselves (see also Chapter 5).

In the last 15 years, the methodical procedure of Intermodal Decentering, which structures the session with clients in a certain way (Section 4.1), has developed with these elements. After a conversation that addresses the concerns and resources (Section 4.3) as well as the ideas about a "good future" (Section 4.4) in a curious and appreciative way, a phase of artistic or playful activity is inserted (Section 4.6). This activity is carefully brought back into language (Section 4.7) and then made available for further work (Section 4.8) and used (Section 4.9). It should be noted that by no means every session we conduct includes a phase of decentering. Decentering in different settings has very specific effects. Therefore, it is advisable to use it in a targeted way (see the comments in Chapter 7).

Artistic activity and language mutually enrich each other in a positive way. The possibilities for reflection are increased by the observable artistic activity, as well as by the contemplation of the work, and lead to new layers. Through the inclusion of the sensory aspect, new dimensions of experience open up, which in turn are deepened and concretized through the appreciative act of being put into words. From a cognitive point of view, one can often observe something like "aha" experiences, which point to possible new perspectives and stimulate new ways and concretizations. The sensory experiences that are less easy to put into words, the experience of mastering an unfamiliar task, and feelings of inner involvement are likely to be at least as meaningful for further positive progress (see our comments on this in Chapter 6).

1.2 Our intended audience

It was the authors' intention and aim to write a textbook that makes the practical process clear in detail, discusses the roots and theoretical framework of the method, and describes the characteristics of the main elements—language, art, and play.

The book is not a self-help book. It is aimed at professionals and those who want to become professionals. The circle of such professionals can be drawn wide. We think of psychologists, therapists, coaches, supervisors, career counselors, educational consultants, and social workers with counseling functions. However, the book should also be helpful to professionals who take on episodic counseling roles—nurses, counselors, nutritionists, physicians, teachers, special and social educators, and others.

Furthermore, the way we approach artistic activity and language should be beneficial almost everywhere in direct interaction with others, at least where it is (also) about personal matters. In Chapter 2, we go into those aspects of our method of working that may be familiar or new to readers coming from other backgrounds and that should be taken into account. In Chapters 7 and 9, we discuss the applications and professional requirements in the areas of work in which we have been able to gain experience so far.

Finally, a note on the use of feminine and masculine pronouns within the text. Both authors are men, but the majority of our colleagues and students are female. We have decided to use both forms alternately within sections, which means that one form is sometimes used more frequently than the other.

1.3 Background of the authors

Both authors have been exposed to a wide range of therapeutic and counseling approaches throughout their long professional careers.

Herbert Eberhart, originally coming from psychoanalysis, has theoretically and practically dealt in depth with the different approaches of humanistic psychology in the course of his professional development. He became aware of systems theory as early as the beginning of the 1970s. He was the first to introduce the counseling consequences of this metatheoretical approach into Swiss-German career counseling and social services. He was also the first to propagate and teach the solution-oriented approach to counseling in these two professional fields. In 1998, together with others, he founded the Swiss Network for Solution-Oriented Work. Solution orientation does away with the paradoxical claim that in order to make progress in counseling and therapy, one must have increasingly detailed knowledge of pathology (see also Sections 8.3 and 8.4).

Decades of intensive collaboration with Paolo Knill and the examination of the art-oriented approach to work have led, on the one hand, to the method of Intermodal Decentering and, on the other hand, to a broad, very fundamental view of what happens in counseling and therapy. Herbert Eberhart works as a trainer, coach, supervisor, and short-term therapist in private practice.

Paolo Knill, a natural scientist and musician who only later earned a doctorate in psychology, has always been fascinated by the processes triggered by the inclusion of art with individuals, groups, teams, and large groups. As a junior partner, he gained his first experience in management consulting. As a pioneer of group improvisation, he taught free improvisation at Swiss conservatories, schools for social service work, and in teacher training from 1970. It was in this context that he first exchanged ideas with Herbert Eberhart.

In 1973–74, he was a visiting professor of music education at Tufts University, Medford, Massachusetts. During this decade, he also expanded his expertise in the clinical field. He became one of the founders of music therapy in German-speaking Switzerland. In the context of his therapeutic experiences in psychiatry and private practice, he turned to a phenomenological view of the process of change. On this basis, supplemented by clinical practice and experience in education and counseling, he developed the Intermedial Concept of the Arts in change processes. This became the content of the Expressive Arts Therapy department he co-founded in 1974 at Lesley University, Cambridge, Massachusetts, where Paolo Knill taught as a full professor from 1978 to 1992.

Paolo Knill is the rector of the international university institute European Graduate School in Saas-Fee, Valais (Switzerland). In the department of Art, Health, and Society, the principles presented here are taught and lived. Paolo Knill is active today primarily as an instructor but also as a coach and supervisor.

The numerous cases in our book are not made up but originate from our actual practice. Details have been altered so that clients cannot be identified.

1.4 Getting started at different points as well as cross-reading

The book can be read in the order presented. However, this is by no means a requirement. Those who already feel sufficiently informed by this introduction can begin with the section that best speaks to them.

Experienced practitioners may first want to get an overview of the origin and evolution of our way of working. We then recommend starting with Chapter 2 (The Idea of Going Together) and then reading (parts of) Chapter 8 (The Origins). Here, it becomes clear how close or how far one's thinking and practice are to be positioned in comparison to the presented approach that we are working with.

Suppose you think systemically and are close to the resource and solution orientation but cannot imagine exactly how to incorporate artistic activities into your daily practice. In that case, you could start with Chapter 4 (Section 4.6).

Artists and art therapists might want to orient themselves first with our understanding of artistic activity and, in this case, start with Chapter 5.

1.5 And finally thanks to...

First of all, we would like to thank our current and former students. Their questions, commitment, enthusiasm, and life experiences have always given us food for thought and encouraged us to continue.

We also thank our partners who, time and again, had to be very patient because their husbands were absent in joint retreats or holed up behind the computer.

Last but not least, we would like to thank Maja Loeliger and Barbara Traber, who dealt with our sometimes bumpy language. Further, Dr. Andreas Bürgi, Marie-Louise Ries, and Peter Truniger who took the trouble to comment on the text in a scholarly and critical way. And finally, Günter Presting from the publishing house Vandenhoeck & Ruprecht, who ensured through his suggestions that readers who are less familiar with the subject matter can also find access to our discourse.

What remains

What has remained are the two different worlds: that of the arts and that of applied psychology focused on the counseling and therapeutic process. This difference seems to be a very fundamental one. That is why the language of one cannot simply be translated into the language of the other.

We usually experience this difference not as painful but as enriching. If we are impatient, however, we occasionally experience it as a disturbance and a hindrance. The difference in our understanding of the world and human beings forces us to listen carefully, witness sensitively, and allow the communication process to unfold at a slower pace.

What has remained is the fascination with the unexpected and the moving. We experience it in conversations with our clients, but above all in artistic activity and where art and language meet.

In our work with clients and in our training work, the integration of both worlds is positively responded to throughout. Their difference is moving, affects, opens new perspectives, and leads to surprising shifts, which—although one only notices this later—turn out to be positive and desirable and mostly also lasting.

2

The Idea of Going Together

2.1 Thirty years ago

The setting: a course center in Switzerland. A group of freshmen from a university of applied sciences for social work, accompanied by their psychology lecturer, and a lecturer for music, movement, and media, who are to lead a study week on creativity.

What led from this first encounter to a 30-year collaboration? The former psychology lecturer comments:

> We were (and are) both about the same age. Both interested in natural sciences and convinced that effects in the field of counseling and therapeutic work can be understood not only linearly. At that time, I myself had knowingly nothing to do with art and creativity. I was a trainer and counselor who trusted everyday language. Nevertheless, I was fascinated by the apparent effect of playful artistic activities. I felt this effect in myself and in the students. At times, we were both entirely under the spell of doing things together and were highly enthusiastic.

The former lecturer recounts:

> The characteristic of the encounter at that time was that the shared tradition of scientific thought generated a mutual understanding despite the obvious difference between a reflection grounded in everyday language and the artistic design logic. The complex, surprising, and coincidental fascinated us both. And the openness in the encounter allowed the first thought-provoking impulses for a conceivable method and theory that gives the combination of

everyday language conversation and creative action in processes of change a chance. The challenge posed by the students who were not familiar with creative work and the psychology lecturer had to lead to a method of instruction that incorporated the capabilities of all participants and at the same time still fascinated seasoned designers. In addition, a language had to be found that, free of jargon, remained generally understandable.

Thirty years have passed since then. The discourse at that time, which was mainly psychoanalytic and partly based on learning theory, has been more and more influenced by an attitude nurtured by humanistic psychology, complemented by metatheoretical considerations based on systems theory. The predominantly pathology- and deficit-oriented perspective in the helping professions at that time received competition from the resource- and solution-oriented perspective. At the same time, interest in playful, artistic, and action-focused ways of working was growing in professional circles.

2.2 The obvious

Artistic activity is solution-oriented

As a therapy, the art- and expressiveness-oriented method was close to the traditional deficit- and pathology-oriented methods. However, due to the emphatically phenomenological view of art as a cultural asset (see Section 8.1) and due to the proximity to the body of thought of humanistic psychology, the opening to resource orientation was there from the beginning. Maslow, Rogers, and others included human potential in their considerations at a very early stage. In addition, the closeness to pedagogy and special education, which has existed since the beginning of art and expression therapy, meant that competencies were always addressed in addition to deficits: Rogers' "Learning in Freedom" (1974), Gardner's "Project 0" (1991), and, in Switzerland, Mattmüller (1979).

With the turn to work orientation in 1989, attention was focused on the aesthetic process and the completion of the work. Each work is in itself a unique solution. This experience is evident even in a seemingly untalented client. When he is led to a creation by a professional with low-skill–high-sensitivity, his face takes on color, his eyes light up, and the joy of accomplishment is unmistakable. By "low-skill–high-sensitivity," we mean the methodological concept that deliberately avoids technically demanding tasks and procedures and at the same time combines this with a high degree of sensitivity in dealing with forms, colors, materials, time, space, expression, etc. (see "Low-skill–high-sensitivity" under Section 4.6).

Thus, any perceived inability gives way to joy in the work-creating process and often to surprise and pride in what has been created. Any work-oriented work is thus work on a solution. From this perspective, analogies can also be expected between the process of creating a work and the process of finding a solution, as it is described in solution-oriented counseling and therapy (see Section 8.3).

> Erika chooses the marimba (an instrument with wooden sticks, similar in construction to the xylophone) when I invite her to participate in a musical improvisation.
>
> She immediately tries to play a familiar melody but gives up again, remarking, "I can't do it!" When the counselor asks if she likes the instrument, she answers, "Yes." In response, he suggests thinking not of a melodic performance but of a creation with splashes of color and listening only to individual sounds that can be produced by different types of beating with different mallets, individually or together. This listening sensitization motivates exploratory curiosity, and it is noticeable how individual sounds are repeated until relaxation appears on the client's face, as if something satisfying has been accomplished. "Have you found some shaping or defining tonal qualities or sounds?" the counselor asks. After answering in the affirmative, she accepts the invitation to do a short timbre improvisation. After the first attempt, she appears to be very satisfied with the beginning, but she finds the later progress discouraging since it "didn't turn out as I imagined." The counselor learns that she was surprised by the sounds at the beginning and reacted spontaneously to hearing them with the beaters. He asks her to stay with this attitude now and let the arc of the whole develop from listening and the interaction of instrument and hands. Interestingly, an arc of timbre now emerges more and more, from delicate brightness to a dense, dark wood sound, which again dissolves into individual high notes—a timbre melody, so to speak. The more this arc

becomes clear, the more Erika "gets into the fire" and finally says, "I've got it, I've got something like a melody!" What she was striving for at the beginning, with the idea of melody that she had brought with her and which was suffocating in the impasse of inability, has thus found a solution on a completely different path.

Solutions are possible even with little or limited resources

From the tradition of the arts, we can learn that art always has to deal with limited resources. Every work has spatial-temporal limits and restrictions due to material, structure, and more. This can be experienced very differently by the artist: as painful, as a challenge, or as a relief. Examples are black-and-white photography, shadow theater, limitations in range or timbre by a musical instrument, the dance representation of a bird's flight, and the human body's limitations.

For its part, the solution-oriented counseling and therapy method points out that there is no problem without a solution and that, in principle, resources can be found in every situation. The counseling approach on which this book is based is strongly influenced by the conversational approach in the traditional solution-oriented working method. However, for some years now, we have preferred to use the term "resource orientation" when describing our approach. It is more comprehensive and puts a special emphasis on shaping the relationship.

Changes, surprises, unique moments

Work that is oriented towards solutions draws attention less to regularities and patterns than to changes, exceptions, and uniqueness. Likewise, in the arts, surprises, uniqueness, and difference are paramount. Even in the performing arts, nothing is entirely repeatable in different interpretations (takes). In work orientation and resource orientation, the emphasis is on change. Everything is in flux. In this, both approaches give great importance to small changes. Solution- or resource-oriented practitioners are convinced that small changes can bring about big ones. Even in artistic creation, the small change of one element brings significant changes to the whole work. The strange point of color in a painting, the new word in a poem, or the change of instrument in music can fundamentally change the whole work. This process can be experienced through the senses in the work orientation.

The client as expert and creator

One of the most difficult challenges for counselors who want to work in a resource-oriented way is the basic attitude of accepting the client as the expert for her own life. Only she ultimately knows what is important and meaningful to her. Only she knows her needs, even if she is not yet able to express them in words. This also follows from the view that human systems behave autonomously in certain respects (see Section 6.2). Thus, every human being is an expert in her own affairs. This especially concerns her constructions of reality and the behavioral plans, behaviors, and emotions derived from them.

In artistic activity, the authorship of the creator is never questioned. Open questions to the client can help to guide the work to a point of beauty that is coherent for her and for the moment.

Accordingly, both approaches value the client's autonomy highly and place an unusual amount of trust in her. Dealing with the client as an expert in the resource orientation and as an autonomous creator in the work orientation is both a challenge and a gift for the professional facilitator.

Appreciative curiosity

For professionals, this requires an attitude of appreciation and not knowing. Appreciation applies to the client as an autonomous personality, and not knowing refers to what is central for her. Both together meet in a benevolent curiosity to explore what seems to be self-evident. The work-oriented consultant adopts this attitude not only towards the client but also towards what she has created. Appreciation thus highlights the uniqueness of the creative process and the emerging work. A facilitator does not know where the process will lead or which of the materials and tools provided, proposed structures, or methods will ultimately make the work possible. Nor does she know when the work will be finished or what it will look or sound like. Her benevolent curiosity and attention to what is surprising, perhaps even at times doing and exploring together, support this attitude.

Empowerment to extend the scope

In resource orientation, the focus of counseling and therapy is on what can be changed or on what the client can change himself. The client is approached as an active agent and not as a victim. Existing or imaginable scope for action, thinking, and feeling are in the foreground. In the work orientation, the focus is forced to be on what can be shaped, and one works with the resources of the material and the designer. However, the designing client is not at the mercy of the material and the limitations but is challenged as an acting person to use the scope. The solution orientation and the work orientation thus both work primarily with what is available in the client and within the situation.

They empower him to take action by using existing and/or imaginable extensions of the scope.

Phenomenological attitude

Work orientation and resource orientation have in common the phenomenological attitude towards the person being encountered. The person, the concern, the expressions, the work, what has been created—all this is taken as it appears in the moment of the counseling encounter. The process is understood as a consultative situation for two. This means that the consultant is in the middle of the process with her feelings, associations, and reflections, but without having to bring this into the conversation.

Many counselors find this attitudinal approach difficult because they are used to interpreting something conspicuous first and foremost—that is, to attribute it to so-called deeper structures. They must therefore be asked to remain "on the surface" in their descriptions. This has nothing to do with superficiality but much to do with the effort to stay with the phenomena.

2.3 Differences

Different ways of expression

In contrast to solution- and resource-oriented work, which traditionally uses everyday language and its logic, artistic design in work orientation cultivates many other forms of expression. Relationships can resound in music, text can concretize itself in a picture as a painting, dance can move pictures, and theater can lead scenes to action. This description makes it clear that artistic expression offers a much richer palette of expressive possibilities than everyday language has at its disposal.

Other traditions of thought

This difference is also evident in the solution-oriented and work-oriented discourse. Solution orientation refers to linguistic theories and psychological models. The work-oriented work leans largely on the philosophical traditions of phenomenology and the artistic terminology of the respective medium.

Our understanding of the artistic process is based on Heidegger's view: "The essence of art, in which the work of art and the artist, in particular, are based, is the putting into work of truth" (1960, p.74). "Truth" here refers to the reality that can be experienced in the work and in creation. A reality that belongs to the realm of imagination but which can be witnessed in the waking state and appears materially real.

The philosophical understanding is also based on Gadamer's hermeneutics:

> In the experience of art, it is a matter of learning a specific kind of dwelling in the work of art. It is a dwelling that is apparently distinguished by the fact that it does not become boring. The more we dwell on it, the more speaking, the more varied, the richer it appears. (1977, p.60)

Merleau-Ponty (2001) understands artistic activity as a kind of alternative experience of the world that is reflected in artistic action through the imagination. This experience finds a coherent logic in the work, which, however, is only grasped reflectively after the action.

Another aspect of our understanding is based on the view that art cannot be thought of without society, as expressed in the view of art as a sub-communication system (Krieger, 1997, p.26). In this sense, art is "communal" and permeates the communication process of everyday life.

These four references shed light on the very different tradition of thinking in the field of the arts. The work-oriented approach emerged from art- and expression-therapeutic work. For the phenomenological orientation of this form of therapy and one of its foundations, Daseinsanalysis, the focus is primarily on clarifying the content of the artistic work. This means that content and meaning become central, even though, in the phenomenological tradition, symbols are not interpreted by the therapist. The solution and resource orientation, on the other hand, focuses primarily on change, which is understood as an ongoing learning process. This difference between artistic - and solution-focused therapies is reminiscent of the classic contradiction between psychoanalysis and learning theory. However, as soon as one realizes that both are inconceivable without learning, one finds an underlying common ground.

The condition–consequence structure

People working in art therapy often see themselves as artists. They identify strongly with what is called in this book an "art-analogue attitude." This emphasizes that a work of art ultimately cannot be forced but nevertheless demands full commitment. This basic knowledge contradicts all linear-mechanistic considerations in therapy. The classical solution orientation produces in the methodical procedure in places a mechanistic appearance, without, however, connecting effects linearly with causes. This alleged contradiction can be substantially defused if one considers that both solution orientation and art-analogous art therapies are based in their effect on a condition–consequence structure. Cause–effect thinking, on the other hand, places a particular cause in a linear relationship with a particular effect. In turn, condition–consequence thinking, first described in medicine, emphasizes that given a condition structure, different consequences become possible (Langen, 1973). The connection between condition and consequence thus remains complex and allows only probability statements.

Different focus of attention

People who associate art with something "elevated" might have difficulties with the radical turning of the solution and resource orientation towards everyday life. However, today's understanding of art as a whole is also characterized by an attention to the material, the everyday, and the earthly, which comes close to the solution-oriented attitude. As a generalization, one could say that, for some art-oriented therapists, the solution and resource orientation is not spiritual enough; for others, it is too rationally reductive, while for a third group, it roughly corresponds to their attitude.

The first criticism undoubtedly comes from professionals who understand their work primarily in spiritual terms. They have a tendency to describe concrete situations in generalizing, metaphorical, or abstract terms. In parallel, they have extraordinary difficulty in speaking particularistically and concretely. There is a strong tendency to reduce everything observed to origins, roots, and "nature." This is a form of structural determinism that takes an opposite position to the solution and work orientation. We do perceive a spiritual dimension in our work with clients from time to time, but we rarely talk about it. At the same time, however, we need to remain as concrete as possible with our words on the "surface" of the artistic work and the play.

2.4 Where we are today

The many fundamental similarities between solution and work orientations have led to a method we call Intermodal Decentering. Chapter 4 provides detailed information about the practical process. Relationship building is guided by an attitude analogous to the arts, which, in our understanding, is in many ways identical to what is described in the professional literature as an attitude within solution-oriented or Focus on Solutions work. We prefer the term "resource orientation." This aims more at an orientation towards general strengths, possibilities, opportunities, and resources than the term "solution," which is often understood in a "doer-ish" way.

Based on this resource orientation throughout, a prototypical workflow emerges, which can be summarized as follows. Clarification of the assignment, recording of concern, resources, and a vision of a good outcome or a good future are based on resource-oriented didactics; the actual decentering phase corresponds to an alternative experience of the world, and the analysis of this experience is based on work-oriented didactics. The yield or harvest, which leads back to the everyday situation, is again primarily committed to resource-oriented didactics. Special attention is given to the bridges before and after decentering.

Intermodal Decentering—a hybrid

We consider our methodological approach to be a hybrid in the sense of the postmodern understanding of culture. This means that Intermodal Decentering is neither an eclectic mixture of the solution- or resource-oriented approach and work orientation, nor an integration of the two; rather, it represents something new.

The work-oriented approach can be used on its own in a client situation. A well-guided and assisted work design usually has positive effects, even if clarification of the assignment, clarification of the problem, recording of the vision of the future, and harvesting have not been carried out or have only been carried out in a rudimentary way or have been replaced by other methods of reflection.

For its part, Focus on Solutions therapy and counseling work has been described in the literature many times as a method in its own right. This means that client work carried out in this sense, purely in everyday language, produces positive effects, even if metaphors, poetic expressions, and the like are disregarded and no artistic or playful activity takes place.

Intermodal Decentering builds on the commonalities of both approaches and combines certain methodological parts in an independent sequence. So far, experience shows that the positive effects can be significantly improved as a result.

Further development

The current work in development focuses on the stringency of linguistic process guidance. While the usual counseling settings in individual and group work have been in the foreground so far, now experiences in new settings (e.g., adult education and community work) and other assignment situations (coaching) are also being gained. At the same time, the approach is being differentiated, and relationships to other methods are being clarified in comparison.

The Intermodal Decentering approach is already being cultivated by various professional groups and educational institutions.

2.5 The implications for professionals and diverse approaches

Professionals who want to gain experience with the methods presented in this book in their everyday work must be prepared to work with their clients in a process-oriented way. Our method cannot be applied successfully in a handbook-like manner. It requires—always on the basis of a supportive relationship—a certain degree of trust in the process that develops between the client and the professional individual. Our experience as trainers also shows that this method usually requires a certain friendliness towards making mistakes as well as a friendly attitude and attentiveness towards surprises.

Over the past two decades, we have become more sensitive to the resources and strengths of the people we work with. This in no way means that we disregard the issues and difficulties that are at the forefront of our clients' minds. They receive our appreciative and compassionate attention. However, with persistent kindness, we explore just as thoroughly the resources, strengths, and successes that can be found in every person's life and usually in every situation. This resource-oriented attitude applies both to the conduct of conversations and to the facilitation of artistic activity.

Finally, the professional who wants to use Intermodal Decentering must embark on the adventure of "artistic activity" or—if he or she is familiar with it—on the adventure of "language." For many who have worked exclusively with the medium of language up to now, this can be very unfamiliar at first. It is therefore advisable to proceed slowly and not to overtax oneself. In concrete terms, this means choosing media that are familiar to you from your childhood and youth, or from your private everyday life, and giving uncomplicated instructions. In the artistic or playful activity of the client in the decentering phase—and this must be pointed out again and again—it is not a matter of "right" or "wrong," "good" or "bad," even if the effort for an aesthetically pleasing work guides this activity.

For the client or client group, it is a matter of fully engaging with the "something different." The task of the professional is to facilitate this and to help ensure that neither the doing nor the work that emerges degenerates into something incidental.

Clients, for their part, usually have no trouble with the tasks required of them in the decentering phase, especially if this phase is presented as a "little experiment" and permission is obtained from them beforehand.

Professionals who already work with artistic media need to come to terms with our way of dealing with artistic activity and engage with the medium of language. It is essential to give as much care to dealing with language as to artistic activity. Chapter 5 summarizes the aspects that are important to us in the conduct of the conversation.

We think that there are approaches to the way we work and think about this work that are preferable.

Those who come from systemic practice might have it easier than others in some respects. Below are some of our thoughts on this.

Familiar will be:

- The constructivist thinking that underlies our work. It implies that we do not view different perspectives of the "facts of a matter" as disturbing, but rather as something that enriches and stimulates change.
- The primary concern cannot be to bring about change through direct intervention but rather to shape the counseling and therapy process so that it becomes an environment that nurtures change.
- The knowledge that the professional person cannot stay out of what is happening.
- The knowledge of the peculiarities of the self-organization process. Among other things, it takes place erratically and includes phases of instability, and the nature and timing of changes cannot be predicted with certainty (see also Section 6.3). However, the practical consequences of this knowledge are rarely drawn.
- Last but not least, many systemic practitioners are likely to feel a particular connection and affinity to the playful aspects of our approach.

Unfamiliar may be:

- The explicit attentional focus on what is surprising both in the client's statements and in the shared process.
- The "phenomenological" orientation in the phase we call "aesthetic analysis" (see Section 4.7). Here, we strive for a strict description of the very surface of work and process, knowing that this is ultimately impossible on a constructivist basis.

- The almost complete absence of longer diagnostic sections within the counseling process.

This may be new:

- Stepping out of the counseling process, not as a break to consult with colleagues behind the one-way mirror, for example, as is common in systemic family therapy, but together with the client.
- Engaging in artistic activity and play as "something completely different" rather than, for example, a staging of issues that have come up before.
- Engaging in the discourse within artistic media, for example, using a term like "aesthetic responsibility."

For **those who come from classical, solution-oriented work**, most of the statements made so far probably also apply. In addition, the following can be mentioned.

Familiar will be:

- The nature of conversation in the phases before decentering and in the follow-up phase (Section 4.9).

Unfamiliar may be:

- Engaging in purely associative statements by the client in the "harvesting" phase (Section 4.8).

New might be:

- The way of talking to and accompanying the client during the artistic activity or play in the decentering phase. It can be compared with aspects of the traditional role of a coach in sports ("art coach").

Those who work with artistic media and already use them in their work are also likely to have easier access to our way of working.

Familiar will be:

- The view that human cultural wealth is inconceivable without art and artistic activity, and thus that all people have access in some way to creative agency.
- Artistic activity today, even if practiced in single disciplines, both in the popular and in the actual art business, occurs in mixed media and forms new focal points, such as mixed media, shows, MTV (Music Television), performance art, film, dance theater, etc. Even if an artist has "tuned in" to one genre, so to speak, access to contemporary culture is made easier if he or she gains experience in all art forms. In our work, interdisciplinary training of professionals has a positive effect, as it allows us to better respond to clients' inclinations and preferences.
- Artistic courses of action create scope within limited frameworks. At the same time, they demand innovative interventions that can modify the framework and structure in such a way as to create a unique work in a characteristic style. In this way, the complex interplay of constraints and innovative interventions leads to unique and surprising aesthetic "solutions."
- The work integrated in culture is also autonomous and therefore should be distinguished from the creator of art. This leads us to the consequence that we interpret neither the work nor the artistic process in the sense of a psychogram. We deal exclusively with the work itself and with the way it came to be the work.

Perhaps unusual will be:

- We also want to motivate people who are not interested in art to act in a creative way. In doing so, we do not want to interest them in the "art business" or even teach them aspects of a classical-formal school aesthetic. However, we do want to help them create something that comprehensibly satisfies those present in the here and now. (See the comments on "aesthetic responsibility" in Chapter 4.)

- For this purpose, we do not try to use a particular artistic style developed for counseling or therapy purposes but take the whole spectrum of the contemporary art world as reference. This includes the postmodern hybrid forms with other cultures derived from art ethnology as well as popular traditions such as *Schnitzelbänke* or cartoons.
- Not making an evaluative critique of the work—on the contrary, motivating and challenging the process in the tradition of the studio or atelier with aesthetic interventions in such a way that something surprising emerges.
- The different handling of language, which should be adequate for the areas of counseling and the guidance or accompaniment in the alternative experience of the world. That is, the counselor speaks and acts during the decentering from the traditional role of an "art coach."

New might be:

- Giving as much weight to the language and the way of expressing and asking questions as to the artistic activity.
- It can happen in work with client groups that professionals and amateurs have to work together on the artistic prerequisite. This challenge is feasible if we consider that today whole villages create festivals in a comparable manner.
- Not analyzing joint works of clients according to the relational dynamics that may be visible in them. Nor are joint artistic activities of client and professional organized for this purpose.
- It contradicts our conception of decentering to impose specific materials or structures in order to put a problem on a "solution track." We prefer to let the material and the structure itself act as an artistic challenge (see Section 4.6).

Finally, all those who, as counselors in direct work with people, have remained curious and attentive to the unexpected are likely to have easier access to this form of client work. These colleagues are also likely to have a sense of the sometimes-hidden beauty not only of the work that has emerged in the decentering phase but also of the beauty in the unfolding professional relationship and in the innovative, independent aspects of their dialogue partners' lives that they report.

With the concepts of "surprise" and "beauty," we again approach the phenomenon of "art" on a different path and in an overarching sense. That is, we are close to the subject matter that occupies us in this book.

And what about all the others who do not find themselves in this list of privileged accesses or only at the periphery?

In this extreme case (from the authors' point of view!), these readers put the book away: "There's nothing for me!" However, wherever something from our descriptions and argumentations appeals, we recommend making first attempts with small steps within the framework of one's counseling or therapy model and in appropriate situations. This applies to both the resource-oriented conversation and the use of artistic activity and play.

As a professional, trying something new in the counseling situation depends on temperament, something stimulatingly exciting, or something rather unpleasantly unfamiliar. Whoever attentively observes the client's reactions in such situations and reacts accordingly—perhaps also obtaining permission beforehand "to do something different for a quarter of an hour in the sense of a small experiment"—and pays enough attention to appreciation in the whole process will not be in a position to go wrong. In the vast majority of instances, this individual will have done something that, in one way or another, will have a beneficial effect on the further course of the work with this client.

For all professionals who are using interventions that are new to them for the first time, it is useful to get together with like-minded colleagues. Therefore this address can help:

- https://www.expressivearts.egs.edu/

3

The Extraordinary Experience of (the) World in Counseling and Therapy

3.1 Counseling as a ritual of reconnection—an anthropological view

Anthropologically, every society seems to organize or, in other words, ritualize necessary changes in a culturally embedded way. That is, they are guided within a framework of space and time. One could also say that the spatial-temporal container and accompaniment have an "architecture." Some characteristics are determined by local cultural traditions and others occur cross-culturally. We can distinguish between binding and rebinding rituals.

We know the rituals of initiation or transition in all cultures, in every phase of life from birth to adulthood to death. There are also privileges and sanctions associated with transition and passing or failing. Some of these rituals are, for example:

- a baptism, a funeral
- graduation, entry into a profession, retirement
- a wedding, a celebration of the founding of a company, a milestone anniversary.

These events can be called rituals of binding, as they bind the community members into their new role or situation.

In addition, in all societies there is also a category of rituals that address the discomfort caused by interpersonal inadequacy, failure, alienation, or exclusion. Inclusiveness is disturbed in these situations, and the degree of social bonding loss is influenced by the severity of physical or psychological suffering or the pressure of professional failure. The term "healing ritual" is often applied to this category of accompanied change processes. However, we prefer to speak of rebinding rituals since change processes are often about restoring good professional and social integration, not about healing or even eliminating all disorders.

There are universal characteristics in all the binding rituals. One of them is the practice of temporarily stepping out of everyday reality into a spatially and temporally limited, guided situation. A "called" person, group, or organization is always responsible for this accompaniment and the space. It was only in our current society that the archaic calling became a quality-assured profession. For this stepping out of everyday life, it seems that, also in our culture, an attending professional person is needed:

- confirmation or first communion, bar mitzvah: pastor, priest, rabbi
- examinations: teacher, professor
- conscription: army officer
- determination of death: physician
- therapy and counseling rituals: supervisor, psychotherapist, pastor, psychologist, vocational counselor, etc.

In the case of rebinding rituals, the situation is not quite so clear. But here, too, overarching characteristics can be found that say something about "how it happens"—for example, that they are accompanied. In its cultural entanglement, no ritual associated with an accompanied change process stands alone. It is also subject to change in its historicity. However, if similar features can be described in all accompanied change processes, such "traits," for methodological reasons, must be investigated in counseling and therapy before any comparative study.

This book focuses on art- and play-oriented decentering as the core of our counseling.

It is necessary now to point out what is involved in decentering with a "general how" of such a characteristic of all professionally assisted change processes.

3.2 Things that are common to all professional counseling

The "Notenge" and the lack of scope

Most people who seek help have somehow reached a limit. When the distress, suffering, or pain is so great that one can no longer see one's way forward, formulations such as "being cornered," "stuck," "not knowing a way out," "no longer finding meaning," "being overwhelmed," "being on the edge," "being at a dead end" come up. These are metaphors for narrowness or lack, and an expression of a person having little or no room left for resolution or redemption. But as well as the "too much" of confusion, pain, or distress, there is the "too little," the lack of possibilities. "I'm up to my neck in water" or "I'm fed up" are expressions that belong to such situations. Those seeking help also perceive this "lack of scope" as a personal inability and often experience themselves as inferior. The view of resources that are still available is limited or obscured: "I've tried everything," "It's just not in me." There is often an entanglement between the sense of inability or inferiority and the assumption of what the resource or solution should be: "If there were more jobs, I wouldn't be so down," or "If the boss wasn't on the team, I could give more expression to my anger about the bad news," or "If I wasn't subject to such emotional swings in my relationship, I'd be able to find a job!" Another characteristic of this situation is that language also becomes "tight" and "distressed." It always revolves around the same thing: being "without a way out."

We like to describe this state of tightness or lack with the term *Notenge* or also speak of the area of concern. *Notenge* exists with all or any of the above characteristics, quite independently of their cause (etiology) and the symptoms cited by clients. From the perspective of a fate-imposed distress, those seeking help often hope that someone will step in and, like a *deus ex machina*, resolve the *Notenge* situation for them. When people who are suffering find that they are to blame for their situation, they often long for someone to dive in and rescue them.

The desire for helpful "spirits" to step in is understandable in emergencies in everyday family or work life. Also, the desire for someone to leap to the rescue is comprehensible because of admiration for life savers. These rescuers, after all, jump in and out of disasters at lightning speed, with parachutes, diving gear, and protective suits. We know that victims who are caught up in disasters through no fault of their own often feel guilty as well. The images mentioned above then shape the hopes of these people who have been psychologically pressured and are suffering. They are especially to be found when people in the emergency situation can no longer perceive their own resources: "Why don't you talk to my partner?" However, they are also likely to be heard when there is no room for self-healing: "Why don't you just give me some meds?"

Whoever gets into a *Notenge* is always in a complex situation, where a clear cause always remains a question.

Factors from the social environment and physical, historical, and material circumstances are conditions that can have different consequences for different people in similar situations.

In all cases of psychologically expressing *Notenge*, even in complex condition–consequence structures, the key lies with the help-seeker himself and not with the counselor. The complexity of the difficult situation is not necessarily obvious to the person seeking help. Nevertheless, he is an expert, so to speak, who has had experience with the *Notenge* for a long time, but at the same time is trapped in it and is unable to see clearly and to communicate.

Such a situation requires the counselor to have a different way of entering than "stepping in" or "diving in." Above all, it requires the courage to face the encounter, to venture out of the not knowing and the feelings of powerlessness, with the person seeking help as the "key person" in the complex situation, and to find ways that open up a richer and different language of communication. Such an approach might be called "leaping ahead." *Notenge* has to do with boundedness. Now even the counselor, in his not knowing the complexity of the situation, reaches his limit. Leaping ahead (Boss, 1982, p.73) is thus a courageous leap into the opening that arises when the client turns to him.

In summary, *Notenge* can be seen as a situation with a lack of scope. The narrowed scope of solving behavior also corresponds to the narrowed scope of thinking and the associated poverty of language. This lack of scope is also a situational limitation that prevents further vision. In addition, the view of possible resources is obstructed, and the sensation of incapacity, mentioned above, sets in. The logic of thinking and acting within the *Notenge* is related to everyday life but can no longer cope with everyday life satisfactorily. Seen from the outside, it often has a fantasy character, is narrow and closed, and in extreme cases delusional. It is as if in *Notenge* everything is stuck. Thoughts linguistically always circle around the same thing and become poor. Attempts from the outside to argue helpfully have a lecturing effect, especially when one considers that the sufferers are, so to speak, experts on the problematic situation of their experience.

The experience of (the) world in an extraordinary way and the logic of imagination

It is not surprising, therefore, that all counseling methods employ the method of widening the scope in one way or another. Most professionally guided change processes do so by incorporating realities that we can call imaginative. In doing and perceiving "as if it were like this or different," a window of play opens up to further realms of experience and perspectives. Categories of such imaginative realities are:

- dreaming
- daydreaming, free association
- (wish-oriented) conversational cues along the lines of "What would (or would happen) if...?"
- body language and its imaginative potential
- cognitive forms of exploration (e.g., change of perspective)
- the miracle question
- musical or artistic action or work.

In the following, we use the terms "artistic action" and "artistic activity" to refer to all art disciplines. Likewise, the term "artistic" is distinguished from the fashionable term "creative" because, for example, innovation in the development of weapons could also be called "creative" and because the word "artistic" still resonates with a little of the unplanned, surprising, and purposeless nature of the work that appears, without the weighty term "art" being immediately invoked. At the same time, we are aware that this is by no means the end of the discourse on the nature of the arts and therapy. At best, it is opened here, but it is certainly not the focus of this book.

Entering an imaginative space brings experiences that cannot be conclusively predicted. In dreaming, the phenomenon is most pronounced. You and the sudden and uncontrolled belong to the dream as well as to the phenomena of daydreaming and imaginative envisioning—in the latter, to a somewhat lesser extent.

Artistic activity exists like a bridge between these realities. It has the character of a world in which dreams unfold, but, at the same time, it is present in a material sense. This materiality always includes a framework, a stage, a way of dealing with the limits of the material, time, and space. In artistic activity, these are different depending on the chosen art discipline. In the scenic play of a group, dealing with the condition of the ensemble, the time length of the improvisation, and the possibilities of the scene has different demands compared, for example, with individual work with sound or musical improvisation in pairs. We are faced with a paradox. The necessary de-limiting of the *Notenge* happens, for client and professional accompaniment, through dealing with the "self-evident" limits of artistic activity. These limits are self-evident because the phenomenon of limitation in the arts has become anchored in everyday knowledge. We think, for example, of folk theater, choral singing, black-and-white photography, or the "washboard" (i.e., the use of everyday objects) in folk jazz. The limitation of these materials and their design possibilities in no way hinders the richness of what is shown and its beauty.

In all categories of imagination, the events follow a more or less comprehensible logic, but they happen in a way that is not usual in the everyday world of the client. This expansion of scope—that is, the experience within the imagination and its special meanings—thus becomes an alternative experience of the world. We deliberately do not speak of an alternative world because the experience remains bodily and emotionally in this world and must remain linguistically communicable and comprehensible for this world. A permanent exclusion, a constant "shifting" into an "other," alternative world can lead to loneliness, as is shown in delusional disorders.

The question of what we need in order to venture out of not knowing and powerlessness and to "leap forward" into the small opening beyond the complex situation that shows itself in the client's concern can probably be answered now. We need ways that expand the scope of narrow world experience in such a way that new horizons open up in the counseling encounter. New perspectives that make it possible to be with the world in a comprehensible way. The counselor or therapist is a servant in this courageous leap forward. This widening of the scope happens in the encounter space between the client, the shaping work, and the counselor—with surprising results and unforeseen solutions. The counselor serves this situation in the triangle of client, artwork, and herself with her experience and competence in "jumping ahead" and intervening. He remains open to surprising, not pre-conceived, solutions. Compared to jumping in or out, the solutions are not strategically predetermined.

In jumping ahead, the therapist or counselor, in a sense, goes in and out of this play space with the client. With careful guidance, this in and out not only offers a different experience of this world and what shows up in it, but also becomes a treasure trove of new perspectives and learning experiences when the before is brought into relation with the after.

3.3 Decentering—a step out of the narrowness of the predicament

Art-oriented counseling specializes in artistic action within the imagination categories. Of course, it can also give space to the dream and the areas of the daydream (free imagination). When artistic action is the focus, something "work-like" (hereafter just called "work") will always emerge as well. This is true not only in creating but also for improvisational processes in performing art forms such as music improvisation (jazz, avant-garde, and folk), performance art, dance, and theater improvisation. The work-based method circumscribes a technique of how in improvisational play, through free repetition in the tradition of jazz and the avant-garde, works are created from which a characteristic and identity can be gained so that they also can have names. This representational other, which encounters the client as well as the guide, becomes a challenge and possibility at the same time. Sound pictures, dance improvisation, designed pictures or sculptures, poetry and songs, theater improvisations, etc., all with their own characteristics, emerge.

By taking the leap into the challenge of an artistic task or play, we distance our attention from the problem or concern presented and—this is true for most of our clients—are immediately fascinated by the new challenge when given appropriate guidance. Even if, for the time being, we may still have doubts about our artistic abilities or find the artistic framework and constraints too narrow, such hurdles are surmountable through the special intervention technique "low-skill-high-sensitivity" (see Section 4.6).

By decentering, we mean moving away from the narrowness and poverty of *Notenge* thinking, and often from the deadlocked search for solutions, into the challenge of the surprising, unpredictable conclusiveness of an artistic process or play. Decentering opens up a space for play. This also contains, at its core, restrictive framework conditions in terms of space, time, and material, but since the play or artistic process is consciously chosen with a distance from the subject of concern, it opens the door to innovative experimentation and the fascination of the surprising solution of the *oeuvre*.

The positive effect of such a decentering from the problematic to a challenge of a different kind has been dealt with in various theories.

Watzlawick (Watzlawick *et al.*, 1969) shows that focusing on the problematic is always just more of the same and thus makes the situation worse. It can be assumed that decentering could, in principle, unlock doors that do not present more of the same.

Creativity is defined as a situation in which a person finds a new solution in an old situation by setting aside his or her previous ways of dealing with it or, surprisingly, by reapplying an old solution in a new situation. Both can be understood as decentering. Both show the positive effect through a movement away from problem-bound doing and thinking. Both are taken into account in artistic activity.

Imagination theories refer to a decentering phenomenon. The imagination power decentrates from the logic of reality established by oneself. It is not possible with all centering to control it completely. The three areas, dream, daydream, and art, are different. This decentering can be perceived as a product by all participants at the same time only with the art.

Theories of playing show that play is a phenomenon of decentering from reality in the everyday context (doing-as-if). It decentrates from everyday reality and from the everyday sense of time.

Theories of conflict. The defining feature of conflict is narrowness ("anxiety" comes from "narrowness") as well as the focusing of attention on the conflicting element. Decentering, therefore, means stepping out of the conflict zone and opening up new room for play. When I step out of confinement and into new spaces, there is a good chance that solutions will appear. Why new solutions appear is explained in humanistic psychology in such a way that every human being is always already equipped with the full potential of his or her development possibilities.

3.4 Play and the artistic process

It may be useful to look at the differences between art- or play-oriented decentering and other methods that use alternative world experience in counseling and therapy.

Getting direct access to the world of imaginative experience

The presence of the imagined, the dreamlike, which characterizes the tangible aspect of artistic activity and work, allows both client and guide to have direct access at the same time. Already in the process of making, the emergence is visible and audible, palpable and tangible. In the intervention, we do not depend on the description (interpretation) of the client alone, as is the case in the dream or the free association. (For as we know, every narration—for example, of a daydream—is an interpretation of the client, which does not show us, counselors, the client's imaginary image itself, but activates our own inner image reconstructed after the narration.)

An intervention in musical shaping can arise from the field of tension in the direct perception of both the client and the counselor. One can then explore this field of tension either through responding interpretations more or less oriented to the music or through reinterpretation in explanatory, verbal interpretations. We find the answering interpretation in the phenomenological tradition—for example, the morphology of music therapy (Tüpker, 1988). The explanatory interpretation comes from the psychoanalytic tradition.

The body–soul dimension

Artistic expression belongs to humanity just like language. When we come across traces of humans, we also find their creative works. These are by nature not a symptom of a disorder. They are, so to speak, the companions of every culture.

In all artistic activities, all senses are always engaged. This is done as a self-evident part of the process and always in the context of what is being revealed in the act of creating. There must be more breathing when singing a text than when speaking it. A dance of joy or drumming can be experienced more energetically and bodily than the sentence "I feel joy or power."

Since the body–soul engagement takes place in the service of an artistic shaping or design, it is assigned to the work and not exclusively to the ego; that is, it is in a certain sense ego-distanced. This is an essential difference from therapeutic bodily exercises, which must exclusively serve the person and the ego.

The physical use of movement and the sensitive "being-with-your-senses" in artistic activity always shows itself in perception and expression with physical manifestations. These are different in the art disciplines. The use of the voice and the body in music is fundamentally different from writing and reading a text or playing on stage. And yet they are all part of a body–soul expression.

Interdisciplinarity

These and similar considerations call for an interdisciplinary approach in counseling and therapy. Interdisciplinarity is essentially part of the artistic tradition, and yet it is something independent, comparable to the phenomenon of dance, which is as unimaginable without music as opera is without action and song without poetry!

What happens when a text is sung instead of spoken, when a movement is repeated in rhythm, accompanied by the musical instrument, leading into dance, or when a story, improvised to opera, becomes "corporeal," or a previously designed mask is worn in the play? These are questions that can only be addressed in an interdisciplinary way. Answers to these questions must take into account the counseling or therapeutic encounter, the two-person setting, and the concern and resources.

The choice of the creative medium must be made on the client's behalf. In addition to professional qualifications, this requires a certain breadth of artistic skills from the facilitator in order to be able to meet the client in a motivating way. This breadth also corresponds to the intermedial connections of our time, which combine intercultural diversity in hybrid forms. Performance art, musical theater, MTV, and many other combinations of all kinds can be found in the contemporary art scene.

Intervention in the shaping process

Interventions are possible on two levels. On the one hand, they take place within the relational event because the basis of every artistic activity in counseling or therapy is a carefully observed relationship. Relationship turbulences of any kind are looked at. The rebellious, loud anger of an otherwise shy, quiet child against a play suggestion, for example, is an opportunity, a therapeutic resource. The queasy feeling in me, as a musician, when the dancing client finds my music awful requires closer attention in the next supervision session.

However, there is also the second level of intervention to be considered. It arises in the "representational" reality of the spatial–temporal and material design. Precisely because of this complexity, the reference to reality offers many possibilities of leaping forward—for example, in designing, encouraging the client to explore through an instrument, use more space in dance, or use the voice in music improvisation.

For example, a client was improvising on the balafon, got "stuck," and looked questioning. The facilitator said, "Listen to that last sound until it answers itself." That worked. When the improvisation found a meaningful form in repetition, the client said after feedback, "That's it exactly; I just want to listen and feel more now before I talk myself into a dead end."

Intervention on the workpiece

Artistic activity is always tied to the becoming and/or completion of a work. Counseling and therapy depend on this reality if they want to have a lasting effect. The reference to reality happens in the differentiations between consulting space, studio space, and the everyday world—for example, in the differentiation between the world of music, stage, or song and everyday reality.

Here, the artistic traditions offer tools to give the imagination room to maneuver without the "theatrical" action having literal consequences. A fire in a painting does not call for firefighting, and the temperature in the room does not rise. A lament does not literally "accuse" someone, and a "contrapunctuated" duet does not demand arbitration of a contradiction between the musicians. Murder in the musical leaves the dying singer unharmed. The reality of experience, however, is real, is effective in space.

This distinction between levels can be easily derived from everyday theory based on the concrete that can be observed. In the musical or theater, we have the stage as a frame; in music improvisation, the time and/or the rhythmic and instrumental structure; in painting, the canvas; in writing, the sheet of paper or the text type. Artistic play, therefore, gives security and confidence in relation to topics that are difficult in content. The artistic play discipline is, so to speak, an anchor of hope, which can allow the act of distancing from one's own destiny. Each work belongs to a family of work traditions (lamentation, hymn, ballad, prayer, blues variation, dance music, meditation, praise song, still life, portrait, color play, fairy tale, tragedy, etc.).

As creators or people who make music, we serve the work and are not its statement, which is most evident in a musical or theater. As an actor, I serve a role on stage; it does not bear my name. Al Pacino did not evolve as a person from a police informer to a general, to Richard III, and then to an Italian *Nonno*; he serves these roles in the way that a sober choir can sing drinking songs.

The phenomenon of distancing from the purely personal, which happens through the cultural integration of the works, becomes an essential part of the interpretation. The artistic work is then not a psychogram of the client that allows an analysis of his pathology or his problem, but a messenger, so to speak, that is anchored in our culture, wants to enter into dialogue with us, and speaks out in a reflection. Of course, the work originated with its creator and has, in a sense, something unique to say to him as well, but the work always has as many other surprising and different things to say as there are different viewers and listeners.

Personal empowerment and situational mastery within the piece

As mentioned, *Notenge* is characterized by situational limitation and the experience of individual incapacity. A literal physical and mental empowerment experience always results from art-oriented work, and this is within a limited and constrained situation. It is one of the fundamental methods of art-oriented counseling and all artistic therapies that they enable people who do not feel capable of creating and who resist limitations at first to succeed. Such an experience often makes one moved and deeply touched. The person has experienced something that contradicts his or her previous view ("I can't do music" or "I can't paint"), and has additionally managed the situation with limited resources (e.g., playing only with timbres or painting only with two colors). And a coherent work has been created. The success is rewarded by beauty, an "aha" of an aesthetic resonance. The content is very much significant, but it must not be forgotten that the learning experience of empowerment and situational mastery can be experienced directly, is sensory, and is usually evident in the mood and tone of the client.

In terms of learning theory, this coping process could also be seen as an exercise or retreat in coping with reality. In the systemic context, it is possibly a disturbance. And the dissonant belief that has been shaken could lead to new insight through self-organization.

Counselors and therapists who are close to the cognitive schools also see here the possibility of questioning certain beliefs of the client (such as "I am always afraid" or "I can't do anything") in their generality.

However, work- and play-oriented counseling involves many more levels than just the logical–argumentative:

- It is repetitive, rich practice with a repeated sense of achievement.
- It runs on the concrete level of experience (physical and emotional), not just logical–argumentative.
- In addition, there is the sensorial experience: it touches me, it pleases me, my senses are addressed (transferred: it is meaningful), it serves in its beauty to find meaning. One could speak metaphorically of soul nurturance.
- Beauty is a motivational effect. With cognitive intervention, one can feel stupid or guilty afterward ("being found out as if by Sherlock Holmes").
- Work-related activities are a repeatable experience of overcoming challenges that one was convinced initially were

insurmountable. There is the opportunity to create something that pleases oneself and others, and also to contribute to the beautification of the world, which in turn benefits oneself. Therefore, in terms of learning theory, it can also be understood as a learning process with aesthetic rewards.

- The client can have an experience in a protected space that allows the question "Can this have anything to do with the situation in life?" It is thus also a playing field in which inquiry-based guidance leads the client to discovery. Discovery is one of the most fundamental sensorimotor-cognitive learning experiences.

The expansion of the scope

Every doing-as-if has a spatial and temporal dimension. The associated "magic words" or "magic actions," from the childhood "You be a tiger now!" to the exclamation "Shut up!" or the striking of a bell by the person leading the play, give a clear distinction between the play space narrowly defined by literal reality in the everyday context and the play space open to imagination in the play.

It is not surprising that expanding through imaginative play is used in many counseling and therapy methods. The methods close to systems theory, for example, see in the "disturbance" by an extension of the scope of play an "enrichment" (new fields of perception and action), which at the same time can cause a stabilization. If this enrichment primarily emphasizes the problematic issue, however, it can trigger an anxiety barrier, which may be a contraindication. In decentering, the problematic theme is entered into the play only carefully or not at all. The "enrichment" is, therefore, more easily mastered and can lead to solutions in a "phase transition" (Knill, 2004, p.277).

Play range expansions have the characteristics of free play (from object play to free association) or play with rules or rituals (from betting to lining up according to specific rules) and the play discipline of the arts (with traditional or newly invented frameworks). The question of why in therapy with children (non-directive play therapy) free play is practiced relatively undisputedly by all schools of therapy in a similar way, while free play with adults is not widely used, demands an answer.

To discuss the question, we need to compare the characteristics of children's play with those of adult play.

Children have a natural approach to magic and enchantment. They can perform a scene or role with one sentence, often without a formal stage and almost without props: "You be the father now!" "I'll be drunk now!" Adults have lost this naivety and innocence, especially with life issues. It is therefore not surprising that play range expansions for adults are formally ritualized. For this purpose, the play discipline of art and object play is suitable since they give clear temporal and spatial frames for distinguishing realities.

3.5 General considerations of our practice

Epistemological aspects

The starting point of our counseling/therapeutic work is the assumption that the unified world outside of us, the one objective reality, does not exist. Rather, the individual's picture of the world develops in a constructive process of cognition. Accordingly, what is taken for granted as the reality in everyday life cannot be seen in isolation from the perceiving, interpreting individual who communicates himself through binding languages. According to this understanding, there is no objective point of view detached from the observer. This applies to our everyday experiences, our views of the world and of human beings, as well as to scientific knowledge or aesthetic experiences. We do not discover an existing world, but we are in and of this world and develop worldviews within the framework of our cultural involvement. In this sense, we also continuously reinvent ourselves in our narratives. These remarks are borrowed from the epistemological position of social constructivism (cf. Gergen, 2002).

With this epistemological approach, no absolute claim of truth or validity can be made for a particular worldview, ideology, science, or personal view of things. We criticize the idea of a so-called "world formula" of strict structuralism. We attach great importance to the human existential, which is expressed in the beauty of multiple stories that repeatedly order the chaotic (see also Kriz, 1997a).

Incidentally, the legal term "truth" is a construct to circumscribe a set of factual elements.

In practice, the following distinction of realities has proven useful for our work.

Literal reality. By this, we understand those constructions of reality that have their origin in experiences and in the conversation of the everyday world. In the usual understanding of the world, this concept is considered to be the reality. It is usually referred to as reality.

Imaginary reality. Imaginary realities are spoken of when imagined, fantasized, and dreamed worlds, events, or behaviors appear. These can occur spontaneously or be actively stimulated/instructed, for example, by means of fantasy journeys, plays, rituals, images, etc.

Literal and imaginary parts usually interpenetrate each other to different degrees in constructions of reality.

Perspectives of realities. Individual realities in the constructivist sense can be constructed from different locations. According to this understanding, the one reality disappears, and different perspectives or versions of reality take its place. None of these perspectives can claim primacy; each understanding of reality has only relative validity.

Realities have effects; they are experienced. We use the term "experience" to describe the individual content of experience that appears in the context. Experience is our collective term for thinking, feeling, bodily sensation, perceiving, remembering, etc., related to the individual human being. Experiences are context-dependent.

From the extraordinary context of counseling to the alternative context of decentering

Different realities can be distinguished in the course of a session. By going into professional counseling, clients come from a reality of everyday life into an extraordinary context of reality. For the structure of the session, which works with Intermodal Decentering, it is specific that in this extraordinary context, a special zone is established, in which artistic activity and/or play can be prepared, performed, presented, and reflected. The experiential content of this part of the session is what we call alternative world experience. It is a reality in the alternative context. This experience in the alternative context is made with body and soul.

For Merleau-Ponty (Jacoby, 2003, p.112), this artistic or playful experience is characterized by an aesthetic logic. It manifests itself in artistic action and is comprehensible and artistically "meaningful" ("full of the senses")—namely, full of sensorial experience. It differs from the usual reflective logic of everyday life. The aesthetic logic can be reflected and can complement or change the thinking and acting in the everyday context.

The connection of realities requires careful bridging in the transitions from one context to another: on the one hand, so as not to lose what has been gained in the alternative context in terms of meaning-making experiences and reflections, and, on the other hand, so as not to let the lack of mobility in the *Notenge* appear superficial in the extraordinary context of the session.

In order to do theoretical justice to this complexity in the dynamics of the relationship between client, counselor/therapist, and artistic work or play, we attempt to define it through three parts.

The medium includes everything that is used as a means by the counselor/therapist in contact with his client. For example, the communication medium used (language, gesture, visualization, etc.), the materials and tools provided, the specific focus of attention, and more. Characteristic of the medium is that it is largely analyzable, describable, and reproducible.

The immediate is that which arises in between, emerges, makes itself visible, withdraws, conceals, and initiates. For example, the emerging and concealing nature of the relationship, the emerging and receding trust, the becoming visible of a hidden connection. Characteristically, the immediate is predictable, analyzable, comparable, and describable, but largely uncontrollable. The immediate is subject to distortions due to the interdependence of the participants and is therefore difficult to reproduce.

However, in this in-between, something still arises that eludes the medium and the immediate, that joins the two, meeting as a third, so to speak. It is in itself non-transmittable.

The non-transmittable. "The third" is an unexpected element that emerges during the counseling or therapeutic relationship, which is unpredictable, unique, and unrepeatable. It cannot be transmitted but rather arrives unexpectedly between the two parties of the encounter. The third itself is hardly definable. In retrospect, however, the event of the third is describable and comparable. Certain conditions, which can lead to the event, are also definable, but never the logic of the compelling occurrence of the third. We know similar phenomena of uncertainty and vagueness with respect to the comprehension of appearing and occurring events in the natural sciences. Heisenberg describes them as the uncertainty principle, and Eddington speaks of the event theorem[1] (Knill, 1990a, p.33).

3.6 Relationship as the foundation

The shaping of the relationship plays a prominent role in the methodological approach described here. It is true that attention to the architecture—that is, the structure of a session—is essential to us, as is the use of appropriate methodological tools. However, it seems to us that even more critical for the outcome of a counseling or therapy session is the way in which the counselor succeeds in shaping the relationship under the specific circumstances.

Art analogy

Our fundamental considerations are guided by the conviction that the shaping of a professional counseling relationship can be understood as analogous to an artistic process. We, therefore, speak of an art-analog process.

This analogy was initially prompted by the use of artistic means within therapy and counseling. It is theoretically supported by considerations of processes and developmental trajectories as formulated by systems theory.

This points out that a linear description based on isolated cause–effect processes does not do justice to the developments in complex systems. On the contrary, the observed processes are characterized by changing dynamics, feedback processes, qualitative jumps, and the like, and therefore cannot be predicted in a strict sense (see Kriz, 1997b). It can happen, for example, that the qualitative behavior of a system changes abruptly. This is possible even in the case of only a minor

1 The event theorem refers to the phenomenon that events are not necessarily subject to causal regularities and cannot be causally forced either.

change of an (albeit significant) environmental aspect, namely when the system itself is in an unstable state (Haken, 2004). Such processes have been described and theoretically justified until now mainly in physics, especially in synergetics (Haken, 1995). However, there are good reasons—and initial research results confirm this—to postulate the validity of this model also for many processes between or within biological, psychological, and social systems (Tschacher, 2004; Haken and Schiepek, 2006).

If we now return to the counseling context, there is no doubt that the emerging relationship is shaped by the attitude of the professional individual. However, it is always based on reciprocity and can never be defined, influenced, or even determined unilaterally—for example, solely by the counselor.

To stay with the metaphor, we expect the counselor to have an attitude in analogy to art. This means that what emerges between her and her client should develop into something like a work of art. Counseling is thus understood as a work to be created together. Similar to the process of creating a work of art, the experience, skill, discipline, and technique of the persons creating the art are important. However, these alone do not guarantee success. Something additional is needed, something third, non-transmittable, which is not makeable in the usual sense. In the previous section, we have dealt with the conceptualization of this third and its embedding in a general logic.

Analogous to an artist who allows herself to be guided through the developing work in many phases, the consultant follows the unfolding process in her actions and allows herself to be guided by it. This is by no means a renunciation of clear framework conditions, a clear structure of the meeting process, techniques and methods, or overarching objectives. However, it does mean that a high degree of attention is paid to what is happening in the process and that preconceived ideas and objectives can be dropped in favor of something more urgent or surprising. This requires openness, close observation and listening, and a high degree of presence on the part of the consultant. We see these three criteria as central aspects of the design of the work process in therapy and counseling.

Openness and listening closely

We define openness first and foremost as the effort to take the other person as he presents himself. We accept him as an expert on his life experiences. Not necessarily connected with openness, on the other hand, is the approval of the manifested or reported behaviors or acceptance of all the ideas that this person has developed about himself and his life. The counselor, instead, is open to the evolving overall situation and also to herself.

Accurate observation and listening, which could be characterized as active perception, indicates an effort to grasp and describe the other person as carefully as possible. Philosophically, this effort is based on the phenomenological approach to knowledge, without, however, being able to adopt the corresponding philosophical methodology. By "phenomenological approach," we mean the effort to describe the perceived in as undistorted a manner as possible. In concrete terms, this means that we are very attentive to the omnipresent tendency to interpret. We strive to stay "on the surface" of phenomena and to describe them rather than interpret them.

As constructivists, we are aware that this care in description, and the abstinence from all forms of interpretation, cannot guarantee the "correctness" of what is observed in this way. From the overabundance of sensory impressions in a counseling situation, the counselors perceive only what attracts their attention and what makes a difference in their view. Thus, only what is visible from the respective point of view and audible from the respective position becomes perceptible. Perceptible, moreover, is usually only what the other person shows us. And finally, only that can be described which we can recognize with our individual cognitive ability and for which we have words. All these limitations are unavoidable.

But close observation also has to do with nuance—with what one might call perceiving with a wide-angle lens and with the quality of matter-of-factness; this pleads for an effort to describe perceptible phenomena and to separate them from one's own concern or the specific atmosphere in the counseling or therapy room.

Those who observe and listen with subtlety take shades into account and pay attention to the different levels of what is presented. They perceive what changes, often only slightly within a given period of time, and are able to let even seemingly contradictory things stand side by side. The metaphor of the wide-angle lens indicates that it is important also to observe spatial and temporal contextual conditions as far as possible and to include them in the considerations.

The quality of matter-of-factness pleads for an effort to describe real perceptible phenomena and to separate them from one's own concern or the specific atmosphere in the counseling or therapy room.

Presence

The ability to be present is undoubtedly at the heart of the three criteria mentioned above when it comes to establishing a process of engagement. It can be described as an unconditional, focused being there and being present. Also, it might have much in common with the "(hovering) evenly suspended attention" described by Freud a hundred years ago. From our point of view, this is a directed–undirected attention to what is coming from the client to the counselor, coupled with attention to oneself and to what is happening in-between. Brodbeck (1999) has aptly described this attention as "mindfulness."

It is the willingness to be receptive to all impressions from these areas without hastily assessing and sorting them. It is an attitude that does not want to expose or even to lead to a verdict, but rather to explore in a way that is as multilayered and rich as possible. It is the attention of a curious, appreciative, open person and by no means that of a Sherlock Holmes.

Appreciation, non-respect, and friendliness towards surprises

In Chapter 4, a detailed procedure for the counseling session is presented. This is not about a linear, step-by-step process that will lead to a desired result if the rules are followed exactly. Instead, it is about a creative process that is guided by what occurs at each moment in terms of content and form but not necessarily in terms of overall structure. The two aspects of appreciation and surprise play a central role here.

The appreciation, as, for example, described by Rogers (1977), is directed towards the person of the client. It is based on the genuineness and congruence of the counselor and a care for empathetic, accurate understanding. Appreciation is characterized by a warm, accommodating, non-possessive attention that refrains from any hasty judgment or evaluation.

Together with the art-analog attitude, counseling can then lead to what Buber (1962) calls "encounter"—that is, to moments in which it becomes apparent to the persons in conversation "that they [are] addressed on the level of being and that, in the presence of the You, it is about the realization of the I" (Bürgi and Eberhart, 2004, p.57). The above statement hints at the fact that in the encounter understood in this way, a different form of being is experienced than is the case when experiencing another person in the usual interpersonal contact. The immediacy of the encounter creates a special form of presence that opens up the connection to something that could be called "ground of being." In moments of encounter, those involved often feel a deep kinship on an existential level. Moments of encounter have the potency to open up new spaces, which often leads to surprising turns in the counseling process.

Appreciation is for the person of the client and not necessarily for her opinions and reflections. With Cecchin (Cecchin *et al.*, 1993), we advocate that counselors should allow themselves to "non-respectfully or disrespectfully" look at or evaluate a situation differently from how is usual in society and/or natural for the client. This is done in the sense of a trial change of perspective and in no way in the sense of knowing better.

> Andrea, a professional with a considerable amount of experience, is starting out as a counselor after further training in which she is about to graduate and comes for supervision. She describes her work with a somewhat chaotic client who has lots of ideas as a "ride on a roller coaster," in which she feels at the mercy of what is happening—constantly aware that "the track will take a new, unexpected turn." The supervisor takes note of this description but then "disrespectfully" inquires why she was not "thrown off the track." Andrea—after three more "What else?" questions—can name four different points and, after looking at them closely, is amazed at what she had actually done to structure the conversation with her client. After a decentering phase, she differentiates two fundamental sides of her approach (and personality). In her words, these are "the clear" and "the structured" on one side and "the spontaneous" and "the free" on the other. The

same theme shows up in other counseling situations and can be worked on successfully in the following sessions.

Being overly loyal to ideas obstructs the creative discovery that there is room for development. It is only fair that the same attitude of disrespect—and this needs to be emphasized—should also be applied to the consultant's own ideas. This means that the consultant can, in the same way, be "disrespectful" to her own "first impression" of the client, to her initial hypotheses and considerations. That is, she should always be ready to throw them overboard in favor of a new variation for the time being.

Surprises are events that defy expectations and are often experienced as a disturbance. This may also be a reason why some surprising aspects are often overlooked within counseling. Openness to the surprising—indeed, a certain sensitivity and a dedicated focus of attention—plays an important role in the art-analog approach. Coupled with an appreciative curiosity and a climate of not knowing (better), surprises can become turning points in the change process.

These latter two aspects are two additional variables of relationship shaping that deserve specific attention.

Not knowing and appreciative curiosity

The attitude of not knowing has often been reflected upon in the field of Focus on Solutions work. It is based on the expertise of the client, which is particularly emphasized in this approach to work. We discussed it in detail in Section 2.2.

The attitude of not knowing is observed in Intermodal Decentering in all stages of the conversation within the extraordinary experience of the world, as well as in the stage we call "aesthetic analysis." It is additionally supported by social constructivism, by the "Menschenbild" of Humanistic Psychology, and by the conviction that, to speak with Heidegger (1960), artistic activity is an existential of man, which is available to all.

With the expression "appreciative curiosity," we emphasize the desirability of an unbiased, explorative basic attitude, in which the counselor dares to always ask one more question to concretize or enrich what has been described, and thus stimulates the client to enter into the encounter with the other in the same way. This does not take place with the attitude of a detective who tries to bring the client to justice, but with an appreciative, open attitude and making sure that the client never loses face in any way.

Knill uses a metaphor to describe the art-analog relational events between therapist and client as a "dance of exploration and discovery." His co-author speaks of the "blessed artist" or "blessed moment" and thus points to a more spiritual dimension of the relational event as it can be understood in an analogy to art (Eberhart, 2004).

The situation within the initial interview

When establishing a new relationship, two aspects are paramount in the initial interview. First, the counselor must succeed—and, if possible, in the first 15 minutes of the first session, if there are no aggravating circumstances—in giving the client the impression that she is being heard and that she feels understood. In other words, the counselor must behave in such a way that the client can assume that the other person is both willing and able to understand her in her own way. The client, of course, cannot verify this assumption at this early stage; it is based on hope. And yet the counselor's behavior should have been providing signs that nourish this hope.

As a second point, it is vital for the positive outcome of any shorter or longer counseling or therapy process that the client soon gets the impression that the counselor is, in principle, a person who can help to bring about positive changes in problems of the kind that burden the client. This impression may have been already present at the appointment—that is, before the actual start of the first session—but it must be confirmed in the first and subsequent conversations.

According to our experience, it is nourished above all by:

- a consultant attitude that gives the impression of competence
- clearly communicated framework conditions
- behavior on the part of the counselor that appears inviting
- an attitude that conveys to the client that the consultant enjoys her work and has an appetite for it
- a certain degree of equanimity, preferably coupled with warm-hearted humor

- the conviction of the consultant herself that something good will come out of it.

Such attitudes and behaviors are difficult to convey to novices. Fortunately, they are also difficult to imitate, and it is difficult to fool another person in this respect. In our experience, they are closely related to attitudes that one cultivates for oneself as a professional and generally adopts toward other people.

Expertise and cooperation

We understand the counselor as an expert in a process that enables the client to become clear about her resources and her needs and to implement this knowledge in everyday life. She is an expert on the framework of counseling, the process, safety, and appropriate challenges, and she is a guarantee that the client does not lose face in the counseling process. On the other hand, in our approach, she is not an expert on either problems or solutions. On the contrary, she helps the client to discover her existing resources and possibilities and to use them appropriately.

The concept of work described in this book is based on cooperation. Our personal experience and the experience of our supervisory work show that the majority of people who come to any form of counseling or therapy want to cooperate. In other words, they want something good to come out of it for them. However, the way they respond to the counselor's offer of a relationship can vary widely. This offer is not always such that a client can easily go for it. This by no means has to mean that she does not want to cooperate. Each individual—child, adolescent, couple, family—cooperates in his or her own way. It is the counselor's job to "develop the fit"—that is, to find ways of cooperating that fit the unique way in which the client cooperates. This may be particularly difficult in mandated counseling sessions in a more or less coercive context.

However, experience shows that even in such situations, it is by no means impossible to cooperate.

Our approach to the phenomenon of transference

Finally, we should briefly mention a relationship phenomenon that is often mentioned, especially in the therapeutic context, where it is dealt with under the terms "transference" and "countertransference." It is about behaviors and emotional reactions that stand out as exaggerated and inappropriate in comparison to the other behavior of the person in question. In the psychoanalytic model of thinking, these are replicas or re-enactments of emotions and fantasies from childhood, which at the time were directed at another reference person. In psychoanalytic therapy, transference phenomena occupy a central place and are encouraged explicitly because they are powerful tools for the analysis.

In our approach, these phenomena are much rarer. We do not pay special attention to lighter forms of transference. Positive forms (e.g., raving about the counselor) can be allowed for some time, with the advantage of always pointing out self-responsibility and also possible disappointment. If adverse reactions have a disturbing effect—for example, if a client repeatedly feels criticized or belittled by the counselor—it makes sense to talk about this in the form of *metacommunication.*

Metacommunication is especially recommended for all pronounced forms of so-called countertransference—that is, for exaggerated reactions of the counselor to the client. Countertransference can be suspected, for example, when a counselor feels pressured to help a particular client concretely and effectively in this one session at all costs, taking all personal responsibility away from her. Of course, countertransference phenomena may also be suspected in cases of conspicuous aversion to a person or group of persons. Supervision sessions or intervision groups prove to be particularly helpful in such cases.

In summary, we can describe the art-analog relationship as a non-linear process that is characterized by openness to surprises and "the third." The behavior of the consultant is characterized by presence, appreciative curiosity, and an attitude of not knowing (better). She is an expert in shaping the process, provides safety in the artistic phase, and is generally a discreetly working animating facilitator. She works on the "work of art" of the relationship and the joint problem-solving in the knowledge that success is ultimately not feasible by following recipes. On the other hand, a disciplined attitude of openness for "what arrives," which can also be understood as a gift, seems central to us.

4

The Actual Process of a Session

4.1 The architecture of the counseling session

Building a session flow that takes into account the distinctions of the context and gives adequate space to Intermodal Decentering requires careful management of time and space.

Table 4.1 Schematic of a sequence of a session with decentering

Client in everyday life	*Notenge* In the everyday context before the session	
Extraordinary context Concern	*Recording of the concern* Brief description of the present situation Future vision and good outcome of the session	
Bridge to decentering	Introduction to decentering/entry into the alternative context	
Intermodal Decentering Space/zone of the alternative context	Art- or play-oriented design of a work/play	Decentering
Still in the space or zone of the alternative context	Aesthetic analysis of the work and the process	

Bridge back to the extraordinary context	Leaving the alternative context	
Harvest Extraordinary context Farewell Client in everyday life	Back to the concern Establish possible links between decentering and concern Evaluation/selection Reflections on concretization in everyday life and eventual assignments	
	Client in the everyday context	

It is advisable if the phases follow a time frame and certain parts of the process are also clearly separated spatially. Often, too much time is spent in the first phase when discussing the concern. In this context, it is helpful if we take to heart statements that indicate that it is more critical to competently accompany the process of change for counselors and therapists than to devote extensive time to analyzing the content of a problem. Such statements are justified with the indication that circling around problem narratives narrows the interpretation and understanding space and hardly allows any more alternative actions. It always leads to the same thing.

The competent accompanying of the change process, on the other hand, opens the view for alternative narratives and allows for new perspectives, ideas, and ways of seeing and acting (Kriz, 1997a, p.56). This opening of the view is supported and expanded to a considerable degree by Intermodal Decentering. The same applies to the phase we call "harvesting," where, in going back to the concern, there is again the danger of synthesizing a substantive solution at the expense of time, at the expense of competently accompanying the change process of self-organization that has already been initiated in decentering.

To better understand the schematic and to illustrate it, here is a detailed description of a session with decentering.

COACHING SESSION WITH HORTENSE— "GOING INWARD" AND "BEYOND"

Hortense met the counselor at an evening event of a professional association, where he lectured on the implementation of artistic and playful elements in everyday counseling. She is herself a very experienced counselor who has worked for many years in a large Swiss counseling institution.

Hortense requests a coaching appointment by e-mail. She justifies this request by saying that she has been looking for a "slightly different professional world" for "quite some time," but that she "keeps going round in circles." At the same time, she would like to get to know the counselor and his approach better.

Hortense is a petite, lively woman in her fifties. She seems active, open, and curious. After sharing some impressions of the event they experienced together, the counselor takes words of the concern formulated in the e-mail (transition to the extraordinary context of counseling) and asks for details.

Capturing concerns, worries, and resources

Hortense shares that she has wanted to "change careers basically" for the past ten years. "And nothing has happened!" She describes some of her efforts and "attempts," and the counselor is struck by the rather harsh, negative tone with which she talks about herself and her fruitless attempts. He would like to provide a counterbalance for this.

Counselor: "You must have good reasons for not getting ahead despite your best efforts!" Hortense: "Yes. It's the people, the clients, who are holding me back in the current position." Counselor: "What is it exactly?" Hortense: "They often come without inner reservations. Really want something from me, and I can give them something." Counselor: "Anything else?" Hortense: "I am methodologically free in my work. No one tells me what to do." Counselor: "Is there anything else?" Hortense: "Yes. I can work as a part-time employee and therefore find enough time for my many other interests."

After Hortense has fleshed out her information after further questions, the counselor asks what she has done in the last ten years in terms of continuing education and professional development. It turns out that Hortense was and is very active. She has attended several freely available shorter courses and workshops in the fields of counseling and therapy. She was particularly taken with professional development where music or movement was combined with being a helping practitioner. She has been in a breathing therapy for a long time and has been attending dance training for years where mythology is linked with movement. She also started playing a musical instrument a few years ago and regularly takes music lessons.

Vision of a good future and "good result"

After listing these activities and based on follow-up questions from the counselor, Hortense specifies various details and spontaneously adds: "Most of all, I would like to do something professionally one day where I can pass on something of myself personally in a very concrete way" (vision of a good future). In contrast to the usual procedure, the counselor for once refrains from asking specific questions regarding this point. The conversation so far has made it clear that Hortense has already thought a great deal about the future and, in her eloquent manner, could talk about it for a very long time. It makes little sense at this point in the session to do more of the same.

Counselor: "And for you today, what would be a good outcome? How would you know it was worth coming?" (good outcome question). Hortense responds, "It would be nice to have some pieces of the puzzle come together. I don't mean just rationally, but on an emotional level, almost physically." And after a brief pause, she adds, "And if I can get some feedback from you on how what I'm talking about is resonating." To which the counselor responds, "Anything else?" Hortense says, "It would be nice if I could get to the fears." Counselor: "What do you mean by that?" Hortense: "That I could find a different way to deal with them."

Pause for thought

Here the counselor pauses for a moment to think. Both remain seated quietly.

What should happen next? Discussing the pros and cons of individual options is not appropriate at this early stage. Hortense has already made many quite sensible considerations herself and is "going around in circles." The counselor does not want to approach the subject of fears at the moment. He suspects that it is rather a kind of "psychological conclusion" in the sense of "if I have been working on this for so long, there must be fears behind it." At the moment, there is no sense of fear at all.

A decentering, in other words. Usually, the counselor does not decenter in the first session. He looks at the clock. There are 35 minutes left. That is short, actually too short. But decentering makes sense; it opens up the chance for something more fundamental to come into play. But what to do? The counselor wants to avoid at all costs that Hortense should feel compelled to give a sample of her skills. So anything that has to do with movement or sound is out of the question. It must be something very simple for this very differentiated client: challenge through simplicity! The counselor has made up his mind.

The proposal of decentering and carrying it out

Counselor: "I would like to suggest that we interrupt the session at this point and do something completely different. Will you join in?" (transition to alternative context). Hortense agrees without hesitation. She seems curious. Counselor: "Before that, though, I'd like to ask you if there's anything important that hasn't come up in the conversation so far. Has anything slipped under the table?" Hortense answers in the negative. Counselor: "Now we have to stand up"(bridge between the reality spaces).

The counselor then goes into the next room and gets some white drawing sheets of various sizes and a box of oil pastels. "I would like you to choose from these sheets one that seems appropriate to you." Hortense looks questioningly at the counselor. Counselor: "Yes, I know I haven't said what it's about yet. Nevertheless, I would like you to choose a sheet size that seems appropriate to you at the moment." Hortense takes a large sheet (98 × 69 cm). Counselor: "And now I want you to choose two different colored oil pastels." Hortense takes a cobalt blue and a cadmium green, then looks at the counselor slightly mischievously and asks, "Can't I take a third color?" The counselor laughs and says, "Fine, we'll make an exception for once." Hortense adds vermilion.

Counselor: "Your task is to draw a line with each color. You choose a color and draw the line in one go. It can be as long as you want. But if you stop the movement, the line is finished, and you can't continue with it [the task is supposed to be very simple, yet not trivial]. So you choose the first color, draw a line, then the second color, and so on." Hortense places the large sheet on the parquet floor and kneels in front of it so that the narrow side of the sheet is in front of her. The counselor kneels next to her. Hortense takes the blue chalk, makes movements with it in the air, then starts at the top left of the sheet and draws a curved line across the whole sheet with momentum, ending at the bottom right in ever-smaller circular movements.

Then she takes the green pastel, also starts at the top left, and draws around part of the figure created by the blue line. Finally, she takes the crimson pastel, thinks for a while, and draws an elliptical figure inside the green line, and inside it, very quickly, another ellipse. In doing so, she has broken the rule set by the counselor. Hortense notices the "mistake" and says, "Oh, now I have after all interrupted the line." The two talk about it briefly but do not attach any importance to the matter at the moment.

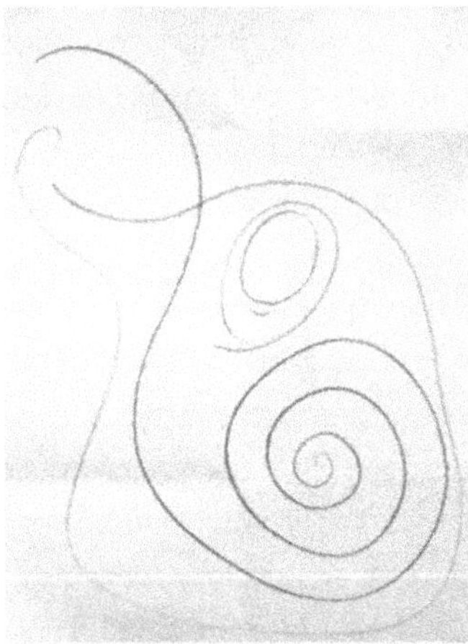

Aesthetic protocol or aesthetic analysis

They both stand up now, look at the sheet from above, and the counselor asks Hortense to walk around the sheet and choose the location where what has emerged shows itself from the best perspective.

They stand side by side at this spot and look appreciatively at the sheet. "It's exciting to see what has come out of this!" says the counselor. Then he begins to ask questions and takes detailed notes on the answers. Counselor: "What do you see?" Hortense: "A kind of vessel. The green line. It encompasses the others—except for one color [meaning blue above]." Counselor: "What else?" Hortense: "The curved lines that come together so organically." Counselor: "Anything else?" Hortense: "They are round shapes." Counselor: "Is there any significance to the fact that there are three colors?" Hortense: "Yes. It makes things blend together. They meander but not into each other. If everything was the same color, it would be more chaotic. Each color is very different from the other." In response to subsequent questions, Hortense speaks of "the depth," the "three-dimensionality," the "liveliness." Counselor: "Is something grabbing your eye? Is something specifically attractive at the moment?" Hortense: "The spiral of blue." Counselor: "What is attractive about it?" Hortense: "There's something very centering about it. It goes to the core." Counselor: "Is there anything else that draws your eye?" Hortense: "The red. Kind of like an egg. Or an eye." Counselor: "What's attractive about it?" Hortense: "The closed thing. It pulsates."

Now the counselor comes to talk about the (in this case, short) process of creation. Counselor: "Did anything surprise you while doing it?" Hortense: "Yes. That I didn't hesitate or think for a second. Just did it. Without any doubt—and I do have many! And now it's good. If I have the security, then it works." Counselor: "What gave security?" Hortense: "It came from you." Counselor: "What was it that felt better?" Hortense: "The instruction. The pressure was then completely gone. It's not like I can paint at all." Counselor: "Anything else?" Hortense: "The colors. That I could choose the colors. Each color somehow leads into a different space. And it does something to you." Counselor: "Did anything make your task more difficult?" Hortense: "No."

At the end of this sequence of the conversation, the counselor asks where Hortense would place the work if something like this became famous in later times. She sees two possibilities. She would either have it massively enlarged so that people could walk the whole of it off. Or she would choose a room in an old house with pastel-colored walls, where the windows connect to the garden. Counselor: "Is there anything else under the table?" (introducing the second "bridge").

Hortense: "It's fascinating that it also still goes outward [meaning the blue above]."

The discussion so far after the decentering action has taken place standing in front of the work lying on the floor. The counselor abstains from any comment. The atmosphere is intense. Hortense is fully present. Comments by the counselor would be distracting.

Harvest

Now, both sit down again on the chairs as at the beginning of the session. Counselor: "Now, if you relate what has emerged there [points to the sheet lying on the floor] and what you said there to all that we discussed earlier, what comes to mind?" (harvest introduction).

Hortense reflects only for a short moment: "The wholeness, the all-embracing." Counselor: "What else? I'll start by listing everything." At this stage of the conversation, the counselor accepts all the ideas without comment and writes them down verbatim.

Any justifications or comments from the client, on the other hand, are postponed for now. Hortense: "The spiral." Counselor: "What else?" More associations follow quite quickly: "The egg pulsating in there. The going inward. But that somewhere it also goes beyond; into space. These three lines do not bother each other. The organic. A certain momentum. The rhythm. It's 'round.'" This is where they both agree to stop for the time being.

The client is now asked to select one or two aspects that interest her most at the moment from the list. In order to be able to do this, she has the noted ideas read to her again slowly. She chooses "going inward" and "beyond" and would like to start with "going inward" for further elaboration.

Counselor: "If this 'going within' is indeed a real reference, what might that mean?" Hortense: "I have started to meditate. It's an inclination I have. It's a little bit at the expense of... [pauses]. No, actually, it's not at any expense." Counselor: "What does that mean specifically?" Hortense: "Really giving me that time." Counselor: "Anything else?" Hortense: "I might be able to guide others to go inward as well."

Regarding the aspect "beyond," the client says that it is important not to simply sink into oneself. Instruction in meditation, in particular, would be a means to avoid this. Going "beyond" is difficult for her and is fraught with fear. She feels insecure. There is definitely not enough time to continue here in more concrete terms.

The counselor concludes this first session. He again mentions the framework conditions of a coaching session (repetition from the e-mail correspondence) and, in accordance with her expressed wish, gives Hortense his preliminary impression of her situation: Hortense gives him the impression of a woman who has done a great deal. She seems very capable of making differentiations and seems to be extremely successful professionally. Her question is very comprehensible to him. From his point of view, it is about something like "the successful life."

Sustainable continuation

Since the work on decentering is not really finished, the counselor gives Hortense "a suggestion" to take with her. She is to bring for the next session on a disk "something where the 'going within' and the 'beyond' come into conversation with each other."

Three weeks later, Hortense brings on a disk a sequence of improvisations she composed on her musical instrument and "worked on for a long time." She worked out both themes for herself alone on the instrument and then brought them "into conversation with each other" in a three-part run-through, with various surprises along the way. Counselor and client rework the work they brought with them with aesthetic analysis and questions about the harvest.

The metaphor of "going within" and "beyond" also accompanies the third session, at which the coaching can be concluded with a preliminary, good result. "The pressure is off" from the initial question. Hortense will do some clarification and has already "picked up the first threads." She has also become aware that the professional world is only a relatively small part of her life. "I will step out with my own... But I will also be stimulated—and have quiet moments. There's a rhythm to everything. There's a time for everything."

4.2 Clarification of assignment

Not seldom do difficult counseling sessions fail because the assignment—or, as it is sometimes called, the work contract—has not been clarified with sufficient care at the beginning of the discussions. This is a general aspect of consulting, which also has its importance in our approach.

Different approaches

At some point during the first session with a client, the way forward must be discussed and agreed upon. Often, certain aspects of a possible agreement have already been discussed during the initial telephone contact. In this case, the counselor can and should refer to this conversation.

What is considered a favorable time for clarifying the assignment within the first session is likely to vary from person to person. Some counselors like to go *in media res* and only come to talk about the possible further work and its manner towards the end of the first session. Others first talk in more detail about the way they work and perhaps also clarify the context of the referral. Third, the whole first session is designed as a clarification session, trying to establish a detailed diagnosis in order to be able to outline a possible work contract based on this.

The approach presented in this book is, to a large extent, process-oriented—that is, the professional is guided by what happens. Thus, she will adapt her approach to the clarification of the assignment to the particular situation and may also tend to do a bit of problem formulation in the first session. This allows both sides to probe whether a promising collaboration can be expected or not.

In supervision and coaching of individual clients, the following process has proven successful in our practice. At the beginning of the first session, the referral context is clarified. After two or three sentences about his way of working, the counselor tries to grasp in broad outline the client's situation and specific concerns. Whenever possible, he then begins to work on a problematic (partial) aspect, with the client's consent.

Such a process provides the client with concrete insight into the counselor's way of working. In the positive case, this also results in a small or even more significant sense of achievement, which inspires further work. It is only towards the end of the first session that we present our working method in more detail, discuss the framework conditions (fee, length, and frequency of sessions, provisional duration of the cooperation), and concretize the details of a possible assignment together with the client. In rare cases, the counselor will give reasons at this time why she is unwilling to accept an assignment and will provide assistance with a referral to a third party if one is desired. As a rule, the client is given time to think about whether or not she wants to engage in a work contract on the terms discussed.

If there is obvious mutual agreement, the assignment is formulated again verbally, and the next meeting date is already fixed. If an institution pays for the counseling, the agreed points are also recorded in writing. The written confirmation of the assignment should also contain information about any obligation to disclose a client's situation.

The approach outlined is suitable for institutions and independent practice where clients voluntarily come to us for somewhat shorter sequences of counseling and therapy. However, the tradition is somewhat different for therapies in the clinical setting or with patients covered by health insurance, which usually last longer. Here, as a rule, the first steps to be taken are those that lead to the diagnosis that justifies the therapy.

Mandated clients

In the case of mandated clients, the situation is different again. Here, there is an authority in the background that has mandated or at least strongly recommended counseling, coaching, supervision, or therapy. This usually results in the counselor appearing to the client, at least initially, as an extension of the institution and therefore being perceived primarily in his controlling function. The fact that a counselor exercises direct or indirect control may make sense in certain situations. For example, he may be obliged to report unexcused absences of the client to the referring authority.

The question of motivation often poses another difficulty for mandated clients. Every professionally guided change process requires an extraordinary commitment from the client. This is no different from the approach presented here. In mandated sessions, the initial situation must be clarified in any case during the initial contact. In our practice, it has proven effective to do this immediately after the warm-up or attunement phase (sometimes called the social phase). We briefly inform the client about what we know from previous contacts, telephone conversations, or the files, and then try to come to a working alliance. We deviate from this process if the client is in an acute crisis or there are other exceptional circumstances.

Three aspects are important to us in the initial phase with mandated clients. First, it is a matter of creating appropriate transparency. We want to avoid becoming "bearers of secrets," of important facts, at all costs, as this could unduly limit us in the further course of the work. Second, we like to clarify the negotiable and non-negotiable aspects of the work we are doing together right at the beginning. And finally, it seems helpful to us if, in such situations, the contours of a working alliance are already visible at the first contact, in which the client's scope for decision-making and the area of absolute discretion are important parts. This is also the case when the counselor is obliged to orient the referring authority on a regular basis (see also Kähler, 1991).

Children and teenagers

Mandated counseling is a special type of counseling when the clients are children or adolescents. Children almost never seek counseling or therapy, and adolescents rarely do so on their own initiative. It is parents, teachers, or institutions that initiate or request such a session. Depending on the initial situation, the first interview is different. In any case, it seems indispensable to us that cooperation with the parents or the responsible parent is discussed. In addition, we refer to the numerous specialist literature (e.g., Steiner and Berg, 2005).

Third-party assignments

The situation with third-party assignments (the coaching assignments by the boss, the supervision assignments by the institution) is different again. As a rule, the institution or the company likely pays for the counseling. If the counseling or coaching has been mandated, the significance of the counseling or coaching for the institution and what kind of feedback is expected must be clarified with the contracting entity. With the client, on the other hand, it must be discussed whether he is willing and feels able to discuss the constellation self-critically and what he hopes to gain from the sessions. Usually, in such situations, the assignment is written down. This is less difficult if the client is motivated primarily by his own initiative and is a self-paying client, or if the use of coaching or supervision is a vested right or a customary right of the employee. In any case, in all such triangular situations, the mandate must be clarified with particular care.

Hidden assignments

In third-party assignments, but also more generally when working with teams, counselors are not infrequently confronted with hidden assignments that occasionally even the client or the team members involved are not fully aware of. Consider, for example, the following. The coaching is supposed to prove that the client is suitable for the position in question—or not suitable.

The team supervision should make visible that the team leader is overstrained in his work. In the case discussions with the team, the personal relationships between the team members should be left out so that animosity or perhaps a romantic relationship between two team members does not come up. Sometimes it is the personality traits of prominent team members that give hidden assignments. For example, the great need for harmony on the part of the most senior person "wants" that everything is done in counseling to promote harmony.

It is always a good idea to keep an eye on the possible existence of covert assignments so that you have the option of addressing them if necessary.

Self-checking

The counselor should clarify with himself, or in open discussion with those involved, which assignments he is willing and able to accept, which he clearly rejects, and which he takes on in a somewhat reformulated manner. In our experience, taking on assignments that make the counselor a bearer of secrets should be avoided at all costs. Being the bearer of a secret is usually stressful. More critical, however, is the fact that it limits the counselor's scope of action. This can go so far that important interventions become impossible, and the counseling fails.

Clarifying the assignment is not only about finding out as carefully as possible what the client expects from the counselor. It is also about the professional making the conditions under which she or her institution works adequately clear. If this reveals major discrepancies with the client's expectations, this forces a negotiation of the conditions under which work can continue. The goal is to arrive at a more or less detailed work contract that is appropriate for the situation. This can be agreed upon in writing, but it is often only verbal. The contract determines the structural framework of further work and at the same time makes the professional authority of the counselor tangible in a good way.

On a completely different level, we should finally refer to a sentence by de Shazer that also guides us in private practice during the phase of clarification of the assignment: "Begin each session in such a way that it could be the last." With this, de Shazer urges counselors to think about the conclusion of the counseling or therapy phase in the very first session and, if necessary, to leave it at one session if the outcome is "good enough." It is clear that there are institutional and other reasons that make it impossible to conclude a counseling session without any consequences, for example, after the very first session.

Nevertheless, the basic attitude behind this proposition seems to us to be very worthy of consideration.

4.3 The concern and the resources

The *Notenge* experienced by the client in the everyday context—that is, the situation of restricted scope of action and thinking—is usually presented as a problem in the extraordinary context of the counseling session. We prefer the term "worry." In this word, from everyday language, there is both the problematic (the sorrow, the fear, the tormenting thoughts) and the concern—that is, the hope (in the sense of wanting to take care, to strive for remedy). In order to strengthen the latter, it is important to address the resources as well, even in the very first phase of the conversation, in which the problem and thus the concern is likely to be the focus. Thus, at the beginning of the initial interview, we are not so much concerned with clarifying the problem as with clarifying the situation, with ascertaining the status with regard to concerns and problems and resources and strengths.

The worry occupies an important place at the beginning of a counseling sequence. People seek counseling because they are dissatisfied or can no longer cope with something.

Something should become different. Not infrequently, this "something" concerns a particular life circumstance or the relationship with someone close to the person or an important person in the professional environment. Sometimes it is also about aspects of one's personality or behavior that are perceived as strange, annoying, or obstructive. Occasionally, the counseling concern relates to something in the future. These people are facing a challenge that they do not feel they can handle on their own, or it is about an imminent danger that needs to be averted.

Often, suffering, worries, and pain are so much in the foreground during the first meeting that the view of what is positive and successful is completely obscured. However, the fact that this person is sitting in front of the counselor testifies that somewhere there is hope that "it" can and will change.

Appreciative empathy and problem trance

It would not occur to any compassionate counselor in our culture not to take seriously a concern that has been expressed, perhaps apart from the few situations where complaints seem massively exaggerated or implausible. However, there is a danger— and it is particularly great among less-experienced counselors—that client and counselor will drown together in misery. Through empathetic questions, all possible aspects of the problem are then explored. In the case of a problem from the field of work, for example, references are made to educational difficulties, inconsistencies in the relationship, the general capacity for enjoyment, and so on. Additional connections to experiences in adolescence or childhood may be sought and are usually found.

If this approach is taken, it may well happen that the client carries a heavier burden of worries out of the counseling room than he brought with him. The conversation has shown him that the problem he has been living with is much more fundamental and profound than he thought. In such situations, we speak of the counselor and client having entered a "problem trance"—a term borrowed from hypnotherapeutic approaches (e.g., Dolan, 1985).

The problem with the problem

In the phase of the assessment of the situation, it is important to take note of the problem in an appreciative manner without falling into a problem trance. It is about taking stock. In a dialogue, the counselor tries to get to the bottom of what moves and worries the client, what causes her concern and anguish. *Relevant here is the client's evaluation of the problematic state.* This sentence must be specially emphasized.

Indeed, almost as great as the danger of the problem trance is the danger that aspects of the problem are not taken seriously or—more rarely—are overemphasized. Because many clients in comparable situations have found this or that to be particularly problematic, it is overlooked that it is different for this one particular client. Such a misjudgment of the situation is particularly obvious if counselors have been in comparable situations themselves. That is why every counselor's repertoire includes a question like "What about this difficult situation is particularly problematic for you now?"

It is important to find out what in particular is problematic for this one person within the overall difficult situation. What is later experienced as a positive change is likely to be measured primarily against this aspect.

Specific descriptions

The goal is to arrive at a description of the problem that is as concrete as possible. Counselors often encounter clients who are content with a more or less blanket designation of the problem. They hear sentences like "I just don't have enough confidence in myself," "I'm just depressed," "I'm at a dead end," "I don't know what to do anymore." Such statements are in some way abstractions and generalizations that must be made specific if one later wants to capture even small changes in a positive direction, or exceptions. It proves useful to ask not only about emotional states and states of mind but also about behaviors: "What specifically happened?" "What was going on inside you?" "What happened next?" "What did you do in the situation?" "How do I have to imagine this in detail?"

Paraphrasing

Describing a problem can hardly ever be accomplished in a single sentence. Novices are often satisfied too early. Either they adopt the client's account too quickly and unquestioningly or, conversely, they try to convince the client of their differing viewpoint. An appreciative, explorative inquiry is desirable. What is sought is a description of the problematic situation that is as concrete as possible. To obtain this, paraphrasing is very useful. From time to time, the counselor summarizes what he has heard in his own words. It proves useful to embed this summary in a question: "Do I understand correctly, you emphasize that...?" "I would like to summarize what I have understood so far in my own words: For you... Is that accurate?"

The format of questions makes it easier for the client to make corrections following the summary—it does not matter whether the counselor has not understood something quite correctly or whether another important aspect has subsequently come to the client's mind. At the end of the situation assessment phase, it may be helpful to summarize the essentials of the problem again in the sense of a balance sheet. Here and there, we ask clients to give the problem a (preliminary) title. It can be even better to give titles or headings to spontaneous solutions (exceptions) instead of the problem; these can be used again later in the course of the counseling as keywords.

The opposite side: problem-free times and situations

In our approach to work, it is important to simultaneously inquire about problem-free times or situations where the burden of the problem is less noticeable. It is a matter of grasping:

- what has remained possible despite all the difficulties within the situation in question
- areas of life that have not been affected by the problem so far
- personality traits that do not let themselves be defeated, that do not give up—what is called resilience.

It is striking how few statements can be found in the literature on these aspects. Resilience—the psychological and physical strength to survive life crises and other severe stresses without long-term impairment—has also been little researched to date. By contrast, we know much about risk factors and vulnerability (the opposite of resilience). This lack of knowledge is also evident in our clients. They are hardly aware of the nature of their resilience and which forms of coping with specific situations prove particularly successful for them. They are, therefore, seldom in a position to make deliberate use of these strengths. It is, therefore, all the more critical that the counselor knows how to draw clients' attention to this through his questions and comments.

The questions that seek to explore this can be asked directly. It is helpful if they arise quasi-spontaneously from the client. Not infrequently, gaps in the content of the conversation can give rise to such a question. Repeatedly, exceptions to the problem state are reported spontaneously without being perceived as such.

Thus, A. reports a lack of assertiveness at work and relates this to situations within the family of his origin, which he describes in detail. It is striking that he does not mention his current family in any way. The corresponding question shows that he can assert himself there without any difficulties.

B. complains that he can hardly enjoy his professional successes, and a little later speaks about the recognition of his achievements in a local club, which he enjoyed greatly.

An important point is that the counselor becomes aware of such a connection in the first place. In addition to direct questions, metaphorical paraphrases have proven useful here.

For example, H. spontaneously refers to a very problematic work situation as a "war zone," which for him is associated with feelings of fear and a tendency to run away. "Are there other areas in your life?" H. answers in the affirmative and refers to two other difficult situations as "crisis areas": "Here you have to go and help."

Even though there is no mention of problem-free zones in this sequence of the conversation, a possible direction of work is already apparent in the problem description phase as a result of the distinction made. It is about turning a "war zone" into a "crisis area." In the work with H., this path was successfully followed.

If a client is very strongly affected emotionally by the description of the problem, an argumentative approach can be taken—after an empathetic acknowledgment of this concern: "If this situation affects you so much, there must be times in your everyday life—experiences or imaginings—where this is quite different. What do such 'islands' look like?"

If the client responds to this choice of words, the counselor can remain entirely on the metaphorical level for a while and have such "islands in the sea of tears" described to him in detail. If imaginative elaboration is possible, he can have them described to him in detail in their colors, moods, smells, with their flowers, animals, etc.

These questions are inspired by the formats of Michael White and David Epston (e.g., 1990), who try to resolve the frequent identification of the problem bearer with his problem ("I am a depressed person") by externalizing the problem—for example, by using the metaphor of land seizure to be interested in how the client succeeded in keeping parts of "his own homeland" free from the flooding by the problem (see also the continuing publications of the last two decades by Dulwich Centre Publications, Adelaide, South Australia).

It is evident that these parts of the conversation—for the time being only metaphorical but nevertheless emotionally very effective—can make clear the relative limitedness of even a severe problem. At the same time, this is likely to awaken the longing to pay more attention to and live the other aspects of life.

The miracle question often used in the Focus on Solutions approach to counseling (e.g., de Jong and Berg, 1998) aims in a similar direction. The client is virtually seduced into hypothetically imagining an everyday life without the problem in question. In this way, ideas and needs become visible that are central to this person in question but which may have little or nothing to do directly with the problems mentioned.

Exceptions

Such an approach is methodologically justified. First, approaches to solutions can be hidden in the statements on such questions. We speak of "exceptions" and give them an important place in our approach to work. Second—and this is perhaps even more important—these questions bring an irritation into the client's problem beliefs. Although it has often not seemed so to him before, he finds himself prompted by such questions to recall situations in which the problem did not show itself in all its severity. Even if he is personally very unsettled by the problem situation, his answers show that there was and is one or another situation where he acts competently, responsibly, and effectively. Such irritating facts prepare the ground for the processing of positive visions of the future as well as for finding solutions following the processing of the decentering experiences (see Sections 4.4 and 4.8).

Our practice shows that the irritation of existing problem beliefs can be intensified by the use of so-called nonverbal means. Simply writing down the various "exceptions" on separate pieces of paper and spreading them out on the table, on the floor, or hanging them on a wall creates a visual impression that can have a lasting effect. This effect is strengthened if an object is chosen for each remembered exception (animal figures, colored marbles, everyday objects, etc.). If these figures or objects are then put together to form an installation that is as aesthetically pleasing as possible, and a small (art)work is created, this not only produces a preliminary sensorial and aesthetic overall picture of what "is all there too," but the process and contemplation of the result not infrequently also gives rise to a longing for these other sides of a person's life.

Every kind of successful artistic creation is connected with a longing that is concrete even when it cannot be put into words.

Do good to yourself

Another question that has proven helpful in our everyday counseling work in connection with the problem description is: "What do you do in such difficult times that is good for you?" Here it is useful not to be content with naming one thing but to pursue with the follow-up question "What else?" The answers point to possibilities that can be revisited in the "harvest" phase of the conversation.

Above all, these possibilities make the person with the problem aware that even in the most difficult situations, he can and indeed does do something that makes sense and is good for him. He is not completely blocked. His hands are not totally tied. It is amazing how easily this knowledge can get away from a person in a problem situation.

The counselor's view of the problem

At the beginning of each initial interview, the focus is on the description of the problem as the client has framed it. The counselor strives to gain an understanding of the situation from the client's perspective, already at this stage emphasizing the most concrete description possible and questioning any sweeping remarks and generalizations. The questions about problem-free periods and resilience also make it clear that the counselor wants to form her own picture of the problem, which does not have to be identical to the client's spontaneous description of the situation.

In the vast majority of cases, this is accepted without further hesitation.

However, in certain situations and especially in certain institutions, clients bring in problem foci, concerns, or questions to which the counselor does not want to be confined. On the other hand, the client is convinced that his view of things is the only correct one and that counseling must therefore be geared to it. We can think, for example, of situations in social work, career counseling, or school psychology. Here, it seems important to us that the counselor also takes his concerns seriously and negotiates the further course of action fairly with the client.

Treating the client as an expert (see Section 8.3) does not mean throwing one's expertise overboard. If a very self-confident young man, who has failed several times in job interviews, wants the career counselor to clarify his interests thoroughly, there is nothing wrong with that. For the counselor, on the other hand, it will be just as important to get a closer look at this man's personality and to bring it up. If this leads to a disagreement about how to proceed, it must be discussed. The counselor must be prepared to at least partially disclose his professional considerations in a non-harming manner without simply retreating to his own expertise. Similarly, the client's considerations must be taken seriously.

The time limitation

A counselor is in a completely different situation when the client's description is overflowing with the most diverse problems. If the description of the problem takes up the whole time of the first session, this is neither useful nor helpful. In such situations, after an initial phase, it is advisable to obtain the client's consent to divide the available time. In principle, even in the very first session, there should be time to work on a problem area. In our work, after a first rudimentary collection of all pending problems, it proves useful to take a closer look at the single most stressful one, including problem-free times and resilience. Then we prefer to work on something that can be addressed promisingly in the first session and brings clear relief for the client.

If this is successful, it supports subsequent work.

For all of the above, the description of the problem or situation as a whole should not take up too much time in the initial consultation. All counselors know that a single conversation lasting an entire counseling session can revolve around the problem alone. This should be avoided under any circumstance. If half of the available time is taken up for this purpose, this seems to us to be an upper limit. It will therefore always be necessary to postpone part of the problem description to a later session. This has to be done so that the client does not lose face in the process. His concern must be taken seriously. But we also want to take his concern to change something within the situation just as seriously. This means that already in the first session, we want to discuss the desired results of the work together and, if possible, take the first steps in this direction.

Different emphasis

The focus of attention in the conversation phase, in which the content is about concerns and resources, will vary. Depending on the situation and the person, the focus of attention is sometimes on behaviors, sometimes on meanings or deep-seated convictions, and sometimes on feelings and states of being.

> An experienced educator and consultant, N. wants supervision because she would like to become more proficient in the way we work, which she learned about in a workshop. In the first session, she reports on mandated counseling of an older teacher who was very conscientious but had caused offense with very entrenched ideas and attitudes.
>
> After the mandated counseling sessions were completed, in N's eyes with only moderate success but to the satisfaction of the agency, the teacher signed up on her own initiative for further counseling sessions with her supervisor.
>
> N. would like to be more successful in the upcoming second series of counseling sessions. The counselor's questions in recording the problem situation focus on descriptions, as concrete as possible, of the previous course of action and its observed or subsequently reported effects on the supervisee. He pays special attention to arrangements that showed positive effects, even if they were only small. Since N. remembers little regarding this aspect, he expands the question: "In general, what worked well in your work so far when it came to changing professional attitudes or ways of working with

clients that had become 'second nature'?" Here the supervisee can cite a few things and discovers that she could use one or two of them in upcoming sessions with this teacher.

One can fundamentally ask to what extent this conversation sequence was a problem situation. The counseling focused on N.'s behavior. Should the demands that N. makes of herself have been targeted much earlier? This was done in the subsequent discussion of the goal visions. There, N.'s level of aspiration proved to be quite appropriate. A later discussion showed that the focus on behaviors had proven successful. N. was able to expand the scope of action in her work with the teacher, which had positive consequences. Thus, within the situation of N., it was quite possible to limit the focus to behaviors, since neither special feelings nor conspicuous convictions of the supervisee were in play.

The team of a socio-educational institution was faced with the task of reducing the employment hours of team members. The management had "generously" left the implementation of this measure to the team itself. The task was complicated by the family situation of one team member and the fact that another team member was undergoing further education, where special demands are placed on accompanying professional activities. In addition, all those involved were desperate for a consensual and "clean" solution.

Although many rational arguments were used to describe the problem, it quickly became apparent that most of those present were emotionally affected. Through his questions and empathy, the counselor gave this concern a lot of space. The fact that an artistic form of expression was chosen during the decentering phase, which made the feeling of togetherness tangible, also proved helpful in finding an amicable solution.

When it comes to questions of team members' employment, rational justifications are rightly in the foreground. However, the emotional level must not be disregarded, especially when cuts are involved. In this case, it proved beneficial to leave enough room for this emotional side. It was important not only that the negative feelings could be expressed, but also that the positive emotionality between the participants could be felt.

In the last example, it is beliefs that are at the center.

> Andrea, who was referred to in Section 3.6, wanted to explore in more depth the two sides she discovered in one of the first supervision sessions—the clear/structured and the spontaneous/free—since she is often unable to bring the two together in concrete counseling situations.
>
> This starting position suggests the focus on inner images, convictions, and beliefs. In order to enrich the conversation on this topic and, if possible, to arrive at further perspectives, the supervisor invites the participants to conduct an experiment. Andrea is to select a suitable piece of music for each of the two sides from her CD collection at home. In the next session, the supervisee brings a piece with many wind instruments for the clear/structured, in which the rhythm is emphasized. For the spontaneous/free, she chooses a kind of meditation music with very melodic, flowing parts.
>
> Against this musical background, a multilayered, differentiated conversation evolves. It proves to be important that the supervisor follows his supervisee in the choice of words. For example, the terms he chooses for the two sides—the straightforward versus the playful—are repeatedly rejected by the supervisee.

It has proven effective to conduct counseling sequences in which convictions are the focus not only in an appreciative/open-minded way but also in a multilayered/vague manner with a broad horizon. Metaphors or artistic forms of expression are very suitable for this.

Boundaries

The dialogue about the worry is a central element of our methodological approach. We try to capture the worries and concerns as concretely as possible in an appreciative way and, above all, to highlight the significance they have for the client. At the same time, we also try to use some of the questions to highlight the client's successful efforts to keep the problem at bay, as well as to make problem-free times visible. The aim is not to illuminate these aspects in minute detail.

These questions are certainly not intended to indirectly tell the client that his problem is not that serious. However, we need to let the "other side of the coin" shine through in this first part of the conversation and thus shake the often very rigid convictions about the problem.

Based on the described approach to the problem, we find ourselves between the positions of the classical solution orientation, which would prefer not to address the problem at all (e.g., de Shazer, 1989a), and the traditional art orientation, which usually tries to capture the problematic situation with all its painful and constricting aspects in great detail both linguistically and artistically (e.g., Levine, 1995).

In contrast to the classical solution orientation, our questions do not focus heavily on the client's behavior. The meanings that the client attributes to his experiences, the underlying narratives, play just as important a role. Equally important are the often very negative feelings associated with the problems. Nevertheless, we do not believe that these feelings should be given special consideration.

In summary, we make sure that every description of a problem addresses both the individual significance of the problematic issue and the abilities, strengths, and resources that are present at the same time. We emphasize the latter through our questions and comments without giving the impression that we are taking the problem less seriously because of this. Even in this phase of the conversation, we usually do not spare compliments, even if they may only be expressed discreetly or indirectly, such as our amazement at what is still possible despite the possibly immense limitations caused by the problem.

The yardstick for the "correctness" of the description of a problem is always how the client experiences what is problematic for him. Arguing or even correcting on the part of the counselor is not appropriate. On the other hand, it is useful to have specific aspects of the problem described as concretely as possible. As has already been pointed out, an interested attitude of not knowing is helpful. However, the counselor's approach to the problem can also include critical questioning. Often the problem then appears in a somewhat different light at the end of the conversational segment.

Taking stock, rather than possible explanations about the origins of problems and difficulties, is central to capturing concern. Depending on the situation and the person, the focus may be on behaviors, feelings, or beliefs. Our experience shows that explanations may be fascinating but contribute little to grasping the overall situation and even less to solutions.

That is because cultural and social components are hidden in many explanations. Social constructivism points out this fact and emphasizes that other, equally plausible explanations are always possible in every situation. In everyday counseling, we take note of explanations but usually do not elaborate on them. We feel supported in this behavior by the psychiatric diagnostic manual *DSM-IV* (Saß *et al.*, 1996), according to which a "diagnosis" is about an inventory of the disorder and not about an etiological statement.

Even in the first session, it makes sense to limit the time taken in the phase of problem and situation assessment. A positive course of the entire counseling or therapy process is more guaranteed if one aspect of the concern can be worked on concretely in the first session than by a comprehensive inventory.

4.4 The vision of a good result

In the past century, the field of psychotherapy in the Western world has been profoundly influenced, first, by the pioneering method of modern psychotherapy, (> *namely*): the psychoanalysis, and, second, by medical thinking. For both, the basic understanding is that it is not the obvious that matters. What is apparent is understood as a symptom—that is, as a sign of or indication of something deeper. We speak of a structuralist worldview. In contrast, we base our approach here on a phenomenological worldview. We try to stay as far as possible on the surface of that which is taking shape.

From the psychoanalytical or medical point of view, it is this deeper cause—the so-called "real" causes—which must be grasped, understood, and eliminated if one wants to solve a psychological problem in the long term. The paths proposed by the proponents of this school of thought to "eliminate" the problems are various. Often, they are very time-consuming.

The method described in our book aims in a different direction. After the general description of the situation, in which the problem or concern has naturally taken a more significant place than the resources, the professional attempts with all due care to find out what ideas exist in the client regarding a problem-free future. This often proves to be a demanding and challenging undertaking. Apart from the fact that the previously described problem will be gone, it is not uncommon for the client to have no other idea. She has already spent hours thinking about how to eliminate the problem.

She would also have a lot to say about the possible causes that have occurred to her so far. On the other hand, she becomes pensive and silent when she is asked to give information about what will happen when the problem is no longer present. People who seek advice are often not able to name the direction in which they want to change. The future lies in the shadow of the problem or is frightening.

Imagining a good future

By asking people to describe a positive future, we open up an imaginative space. This is unusual for many people and may even be repugnant to them under certain circumstances. Some men, for example, think little of such "musings" and "fantasies."

Strict religious believers feel that it is "unseemly" to think concretely about the future. For them, the future is in God's hands alone. Other clients are not used to engaging concretely, seriously, and realistically with an imagined future. Then it may sometimes be helpful to move away from everyday language and instead resort to a metaphor (e.g., describing the landscapes through which the future path will lead and the encounters that might happen along the way), have clients look for a symbol, or choose an artistic design. Towards the end of this section, these possibilities will be discussed in more detail.

It has also proven helpful to pass on the request as an assignment for further concretization of a positive future at home. An example of this is the task of "letting something fall to you" on the way home, on a hike, or at home, which symbolizes an aspect of the positive future. In a modified form, the request could also be to go to a favorite place (the mountain with the view that you particularly like, a certain place by the lake, or your bed) and imagine the vision of a good future there.

In the case of children, preference will generally be given to such forms of describing the future. De Shazer and Berg (e.g., de Jong and Berg, 1998) propose a kind of virtual experiment with the miracle question, a kind of virtual experiment. In our formulation, it reads something like this:

> Now here's a somewhat unusual question: Imagine [pause] that you spend today the way you always do. You go home from work, have dinner...at some point, you go to bed, and at some point, you fall asleep. [Pause.] And in the night, while you are sleeping, a miracle happens [pause] and the problem (that brought you here) is solved. [Pause.] Well, because this happened at night and you were asleep, of course, you can't know that a miracle happened. How will you know in the morning after you wake up, or in the course of the day or week, that indeed a miracle must have happened?

This question, asked at an appropriate time and with appropriate emphasis, transports the client into the world of vision. This question, asked at an appropriate time and with proper emphasis, transports the client into the world of envisioning. The moment for the imagined idea is approaching. Therefore, the answers provoked by the question are usually very concrete and vivid. Therefore, the answers provoked by the question are usually very concrete and vivid.

The answers become richer when good follow-up questions are asked along the lines of:

> How else could you have known? What else could you have known about? What is the impact of this? What does it change? Who will notice first that something must have happened to you without you telling him or her? How will he/she know (if something is no longer there)? What will be there in its place? What will you do instead?

Going into details

Images of the future are compelling when they are as concrete as possible and are described in a sensorial form. It is worth recalling the very numerous research findings on the phenomenon of self-fulfilling prophecy, which have received little notice from the psychological community (Merton, 1995). In general, the more concretely and in detail the future situation can be described, and the more the description is connected with one's behavior, feelings, and considerations, the more "real" it becomes for the experience of the person concerned, and the more it becomes a positive attraction for all steps leading in the corresponding direction.

In this stage of the counseling session, therefore, the aim is to obtain, in a short time, as concrete a description as possible of a future situation in which the problem has either ceased to exist or has become insignificant in some way.

Surprisingly, experience shows that the picture of the future that emerges in the description often has only indirectly something to do with the problem at hand. This often becomes very clear in answers to the miracle question, as the following example illustrates:

> I. works independently on projects in a larger organization with a small team and is also responsible for ensuring that these come to fruition within the organization. She would like to have coaching sessions because, in her opinion, she aligns herself far too much with the interests of others and cannot enjoy the successes of her projects that occur despite everything and are quite common. In her description of the situation "after the miracle," she describes a woman who does not go to work on particularly beautiful days (which for I. is realistic because she does so much overtime) but enjoys being outside in the open air. She feels free, agile, full of energy, and is somewhat louder, bolder, and more unpredictable for others in her dealings with people than she has been used to up to now.
>
> I.'s imagined vision of the future indicates that, for her, the ability to organize her work time is important. Her description is less about changing behavior and conditions at work than about shaping her life in general. In addition, it becomes clear that nature represents a very important resource for I.
>
> All these aspects proved to be important and effective later on. The conversations in the subsequent coaching sessions repeatedly revolved around questions of personal life design. I. began to consider giving up her intrinsically satisfying and interesting job and becoming self-employed, not least because this would allow her to organize her working hours more flexibly. Nature was also increasingly and, above all, more consciously used as a resource.

When people can engage in imagining good futures (plural!), they make visible to the counselor what is essential to them in everyday life. They do not do this in the form of clever or profound thoughts, but in a very concrete, sensorial, and descriptive way, and often without being aware of the full implications of what they are describing in an imaginative way. The relationship of the meaningful thus put into words to the initially expressed concern or problem is often only an indirect one.

This frequently observed fact seems significant to us. The counselor who devotes herself exclusively to the expressed concern or problem and who also directs the formulation of a good result of the counseling entirely to this concern naturally acts reasonably. If she succeeds in doing so, she has done something good. Nevertheless, clients are often only partially satisfied with such results. This circumstance leads representatives of other counseling methods to question the expressed concerns of clients systematically. For example, they try to identify the underlying need situation and use special strategies or test procedures to do so.

The approach presented here is different. It treats the client as an expert on her own life. In doing so, however, the counselor runs the risk of beginning to see the life situation and also the goal visions as narrowly as the client herself does. This danger can be countered in various ways. Concrete questions, for example, encourage the client to look more closely. Open-ended questions or exploratory experiments such as the miracle question, on the other hand, allow aspects to come to the fore that would otherwise not have been discussed. Repeating the "What else?" question three or four times on the same topic forces and encourages people not to settle for an answer too quickly.

Visions of the future make clear what is in store in life and what is part of the quality of life of the person concerned. If taken into account, this is something that contributes a lot to the success of any counseling. In addition, visions of the future often provide clues to resources that might not otherwise have been addressed.

Different time horizons

When asking about the future, it should be noted that the time horizon that can be concretely imagined for a person can vary. An elementary school student in the summer can at best concretely imagine next Christmas; a depressed woman, just the next morning or the next week. Other clients, however, are quite capable of forming detailed and concrete ideas about a situation two or three years hence, or when they have completed their education, or "once the children have left home."

The "good result" question

Following a suggestion by de Shazer (in conversation, 1997), we have made it a habit to ask a question each time about the "good result" of this one session that is currently running. This question reduces the temporal extension of the inquired future and also massively lowers its weight regarding content. Therefore, the question can be answered by almost all adult clients spontaneously or with some thought without further ado. "How will you know at the end of this session that it was worthwhile for you to come here?"

The client who learns that she will have to answer this question in each session usually begins to think concretely about her expectations before the session and practices putting them into concrete words. This is a kind of training or sensitization both for the client's perception of her own needs and expectations and for what can be achieved in a given period of time. At the same time, the client experiences that, with the help of the counselor, she is quite capable of setting goals and achieving them—even in situations that are problematic for her. This, in turn, is something that few would have thought themselves capable of before the counseling.

The question of positive visions for the future is important. Nevertheless, we do not ask it in every session. However, the question about a good outcome of the current session comes up almost every time. Those who regularly work with this question will, first of all, realize with relief that what most clients expect from a session is by no means as exaggerated as one might sometimes think. Not only novices but also experienced counselors are repeatedly put under a lot of pressure by clients in emergencies. Asking for a good outcome in the session usually eases the situation massively. Should a client's demands be exaggerated, a more realistic good result can be negotiated together.

In addition, the articulation of the good outcome gives the session itself a certain direction. All parties know what is to be worked on, and at the end of the session it is possible to look back at what has been achieved. Thus, the articulation of the good outcome gives the work a certain spin towards the result. However, this does not at all mean that the consultant must obsessively adhere to this. Our approach is primarily process-oriented, which means that we let the process guide us, even if the initial articulation of the good outcome remains in the room. It often happens, especially after a decentering phase, that something different is achieved from what was initially stated as an expectation. What is achieved is then usually better and more comprehensive than what was initially formulated. And it is not uncommon for the initially expressed concern to have taken care of itself; occasionally, however, its processing has to be postponed to the next session.

Language well shaped

We have already pointed out that it is crucial to obtain, as far as possible, specific descriptions of what is expected from the counseling session or from a good future. A specific, sensorial description not only facilitates later review but makes ideas about the future truly tangible for the soul's experience.

We, therefore, work with the clients in general on the well-formedness of the language used to describe the future. Well-formedness is demonstrated by the following:

- The future is phrased as specifically as possible.
- Goals are worded in an affirmative, positive manner. Only then can they produce their optimum effect. Negations and comparatives (intensifiers) should be rephrased: "I don't want to experience this fear in situations like this anymore." "What would you like to experience instead of fear?" "I would like to have more courage (comparative)." "Then what are you like when you have 'more courage'?"
- Goals are articulated in such a way that they are within the client's sphere of control and competence and are associated with activity.
- The formulation of a desired future behavior or state always includes indicators and metrics to determine whether or not the desired has occurred: "How will you know that you are facing X clearly?" "How might I notice this as an outside observer?" "What difference will this make from your current behavior?"

In other words, it is about expressing positive visions of the future in detailed, differentiated, rich language. This language should be as concrete and tangible as possible. As a result, it dispenses with the "big" nouns so common in German (e.g., more self-confidence, showing consistency, enjoying freedom) and refrains from platitudes and generalities.

The already visible "tip" of a good future

If the client is able to find situations in her life where this future is already present to some extent, the chance that previously formulated goals and visions of a positive future will be achieved increases significantly. We always focus our attention on this aspect not only when discussing the problem and the counseling issue but also when formulating goals and visions for the future. This means that we pay attention to wherever strengths, abilities, and what has already been achieved become visible, and at the same time, we also make an effort to ask related and appropriate questions. The Focus on Solutions counseling approach speaks in this context of the questions for exceptions.

Other forms of expression

Many clients find it difficult to verbalize visions of the future in relation to themselves. This is especially true when desired attitudes and states of being are in the foreground. It can therefore be both facilitating and clarifying if clients are asked to express what they are striving for in a different form.

> A. is working on a larger consulting team for the first time in her life. She used to run her own dance studio. A. has trouble finding her way around the team situation, even though this may not be readily apparent to outsiders. Most difficult for her are the team meetings. A., who is lively and active in everyday life, becomes quiet here and clearly notices how she becomes physically tense.
>
> From counseling, A. expects impulses so that she can "wake up" in the team. She underlines her report of her situation with a lot of gestures and facial expressions. The counselor asks some concrete questions about the desired "being awake" in upcoming team meetings and then asks A. to make the situation "visible" for him. A. should

first demonstrate to him concretely in posture and movement how she is currently sitting in the team meeting. Then, without speaking or overthinking, she is to find three possible posture or movement forms that express something of her vision of the future. A. does this with a lot of concentration and inner attention.

In this case, the counselor was able to use the client's preferred (physical) form of expression and continue to work directly on this form of expression as the session progressed, without an actual decentering phase in between, in order to open the way to possible solutions.

A. investigates the physical and mental movement and posture requirements for the variations shown and considers whether these forms of physical expression might have something to do with her as a person. At the end of the session, the counselor and A. agree that she will temporarily adopt the postures she has found, as far as possible and appropriate, in the next team session and then observe what happens.

Four weeks later, A. reported striking effects of this experiment. The different postures adopted on a trial basis meant that she spoke up significantly more than in previous sessions. This seemed to irritate some of those present, especially the team leader, but also earned her positive feedback from colleagues. The effects in the following weeks are also noteworthy: her position with other employees has clarified in various ways, which A. sees as positive. The strongest effects are with herself. She feels that she now moves very differently in the team. She no longer feels cold.

A. has also discovered that these postures also have positive effects in her private life, which is often quite tense. She now wants to continue working on this in the follow-up session.

In this particular case, the physical-symbolic expression of goal visions proved to be a medium that could be used directly for finding and later concretizing the solution. This is not often the case. However, the example shows how a counselor can successfully accompany and guide the client as an expert from the attitude of not knowing together with a bodily-sensory expression.

As a rule, the use of symbolic or metaphorical forms of expression to concretize target visions is less spectacular in its effect. The color chosen to represent the atmosphere the supervisee wants to strengthen in her counseling room, the music CD chosen at home to symbolize the envisioned new attitude towards life, or the object that reminds the client of a particular behavior she wants to adopt are all examples of possible nonverbal expressions of what is aspired to or longed for.

In a certain way, the use of such means obscures the precision in language of the vision of a positive future called for in our discussion. At the same time, the sensory concretization gives the aspirational a new significance, which not only contributes to the specification of what is being aspired to but can also support the achievement of the vision or the imagined to a considerable extent.

Ambivalence

In addition to the difficulty of putting visions of goals into words and making them concrete, goal ambivalence can also be observed here and there. The client does not know what she should tackle first or in which direction she would most like to take steps. It is true that the counselor can usually count on a carefully conducted decentering phase to bring clarification. However, the ambivalence expressed in the conversation can be so intense and agonizing that it makes sense to address it immediately.

In such a situation, it is possible to put the problem expressed in the previous phase of the conversation aside for processing and work primarily on clarifying an attractive vision of the future. This requires the client's consent.

We have had good experience with the well-known method of doing-as-if. We assume that the various target visions in question have been achieved—one after the other—and review the effects together: "Let's assume that A. has been achieved, in a comprehensive sense. What then? How do you feel? What are you most pleased about? Is there also something you regret? What has become possible now that was not possible before? How does your partner react?"

We then proceed in the same way with the other target visions. Some clients enter into such future scenarios with pleasure and imagination, and picture the various situations in their minds. For others, such an approach is rather tedious or even annoying. In this case, the counselor should not simply proceed, but rather try, for example, to identify proven procedures in earlier decision-making situations of the client and to consider together with her to what extent these could also be used in the present situation.

Utopic futures

Finally, counselors repeatedly get into trouble when they are confronted with goals that they consider utopian. This happens relatively often in vocational and career counseling, in social work, drug help, and elsewhere. It can be assumed that it only makes sense to work on goals that are within the client's sphere of action. In seemingly utopian goals, if they are meant seriously, there are desires and needs, but often also hidden resources. The task is to determine what these needs are and what the client can do to come a little closer to satisfying them. If the client succeeds in setting out on the path, the target visions will change without the counselor's intervention—and sometimes small miracles can happen along the way.

To sum up, by orienting professional work towards aspired positive futures, we step into an imaginary space. This is done on the basis of a solution- and resource-oriented attitude. We attach importance to clients going into detail when describing their imagined futures and expressing themselves in "well-formed language." Occasionally, however, it is useful to choose other forms of expression instead of linguistic ones and to work with a metaphorical paraphrase or even with an abstract concept (e.g., "freedom"). In terms of content, the target visions, it should be emphasized, are determined by the clients and not by the therapists.

If the professional has objectives in mind because of his position, function, or task, which must be taken into account, the counselor and client must negotiate what is to be worked on. This situation is very common in social work and social pedagogy. We also find it in health-care, educational situations, and other places.

Finally, we would like to strongly emphasize that our way of working is not about the formulation of goals in the traditional sense. Especially for readers who work in supervision or as coaches, this is important to know. In contrast to the world of the workplace, the goals worked out with clients are not specifications that must be achieved in all circumstances. They are visions of a positive future, described as concretely as possible, which provide the direction in which the path is to lead and which are intended to ensure that this goal is attractive and worth striving for.

In the process, goals may change as you progress. Yes, this will even be common. Who will then get upset or annoyed if a more or less pronounced change of direction makes it possible to achieve better goals than those initially planned, or if things fall into one's lap that would have had to be laboriously worked out on the initially planned path?

If visions of goals are worked out and clarified in the way described, they develop forces that can be decisive for achieving what is desired. They also form the prerequisite for sensibly moving on to the alternative reality of a decentering phase.

4.5 Bridging

Once the client's situation and the area of concern and resources have been sufficiently explored, and the good outcome of the session has been formulated—possibly together with visions for the future—the time has come to enter into the alternative context of decentering. In this regard, it depends on the style and practices of the counselors and the time available whether this is begun in the first third of the session or halfway through. In any case, sufficient time must be allowed for decentering and subsequent processing.

We do not perform decentering in every session. However, sufficient attention must always be paid to the transition to the decentering phase, even where it takes very little time. We call this transition a "bridge."

The image of a bridge is very helpful as a metaphor. It lends itself because the decentering literally takes place in another place—that is, in another part of the practice space. In this sense, one must speak of two bridges:

- The first bridge leads from the first part of the conversation about concerns and objectives into the Intermodal

Decentering—that is, from the extraordinary context of the counseling conversation into the zone of an alternative context of reality.
- The second bridge leads after the aesthetic analysis, which still occurs in the "studio part" of the practice room, back to the room of conversation or the extraordinary context of counseling, to the so-called "harvest."

The first bridge

Novices' questions always revolve around the way to introduce this extraordinary context and the so-called correct choice of the artistic medium or play approach, and the role the counselor should take in it.

A common inhibition to cross this bridge is the fear that I, as a counselor, will not meet the willingness to cooperate. Consideration of the following behaviors has been shown to be helpful.

Make it clear during the contract negotiation that one (occasionally) also works with art-oriented means and therefore occasionally interrupts the course of the session. It must be made clear that the method of Intermodal Decentering adheres to concrete known phenomena of counseling but approaches them in a contemporary way out of a new understanding of complex processes. This distinguishes it from "exotic" healing methods. It can sometimes also be helpful to mention the phenomena and principles from other well-known schools that inform our method—for example, the solution focus, the power of imagination, the principle of "no more of the same"; resource orientation, latitude for decision-making, patterns of learning, etc.

At the beginning, invite the client to a "laboratory" or "experiment," which is carefully evaluated afterward and reviewed in the next session. Often it is sufficient to interrupt the session and announce that one would now like to do "something different" for half an hour. The client should be asked if he agrees to this. Perhaps the very first time, it can be added that it will not be anything difficult or embarrassing. Make it clear from the beginning that decentering is possible in a wide variety of forms (artistic, in play); be transparent about what the client is getting involved in before he declares his willingness. This means, for example, as a prerequisite for readiness, briefly outlining the temporal and spatial framework, the type of design, or the play in such a way that the openness with which the process takes place also becomes clear.

Concerning the choice of a suitable medium, we have found it to be of greater importance that the counselor feels comfortable with it and, at the same time, that it offers an excellent opportunity to motivate the client, rather than searching by theory for something that fits in with what has been said before. It is, after all, a decentering of what has taken place so far.

Here, the goal is for the client to get involved and to be drawn in by the proposed activity. This, in turn, is only possible if the supporting professional is also fully engaged in the process and does not casually fall into a routine that no longer allows any surprises for him.

All aspects involved in the choice of the medium or the play process are interdependent and complex, so that it is entirely permissible for a counselor or therapist to develop preferences for certain design techniques. This is on the condition that real decentering is made possible for both participants, client and professional. It is helpful if counselors reflect afterward on the factors that led to the success of decentering according to the following points of view:

- According to the theme that may have influenced the decentering process; according to the experience the client brings with regard to artistic-playful activities; according to the familiarity of the counselor and client with the proposed medium; according to the familiarity of the counselor with the situation addressed in the first part of the interview. (If this situation is related to a problem of the counselor, decentering should be done in a familiar medium that "grabs" both of them. In this case, decentering close to the topic is not advisable, because, otherwise, the counselor runs the risk of not being able to distance herself from the problematic topic even for the time of decentering).
- According to the relationship of material, space, and acoustics as a resource or limitation; according to the time required for a playful activity or a particular artistic practice; according to perceptions and noticeable aspects during the conversation in the sensorimotor or linguistic area such as metaphors. (For

instance, very strong or hardly any movement in gestures or metaphors of speech—"it's like standing still!"—may spark the counselor's curiosity about movement improvisation.)

- According to the importance of the setting (individual, group, or team) and the familiarity with the clientele or the field; according to contract and agreements as well as the introduction of the method.

These types of reflections sharpen the perception of the counseling professional and increase the sensitivity necessary for the choice of an art- or playing-oriented setting.

The second bridge

After the counselor and client are seated back in the original space of the conversation and have returned, so to speak, to the extraordinary context of the counseling session, the "yield" begins in terms of the concern and its resolution. We metaphorically refer to this phase as "harvest." It serves the purpose of allowing the experience of decentering and its aesthetic analysis to affect the concern in all its richness.

It is advantageous not to reduce either this richness or the concern beforehand. A reduction would also limit the possibilities of the interconnections to be discovered.

4.6 Decentering—challenge and motivation

The challenge to step into the alternative context of an art- or play-oriented decentering within the extraordinary context of counseling can only be taken up by clients if we are able to motivate and guide to a "sense-full" result people who are artistically only a little or not at all educated and play-inhibited. Not only with these clients but also with artistically active people, it is helpful to connect where their exploratory curiosity is present as a resource. This is usually the case in creative activities that have not been discouraged by claims of craftsmanship, activities such as building/constructing, designing with clay, paper, found objects, doing-as-if or sound explorations on objects.

On the other hand, design proposals should be anchored in the shared cultural background of client and facilitator so that they cannot be dismissed by the client as "child's play" and the facilitation does not degenerate into a disinterested casualness. Central to the effect of decentering is that client and counselor are fully involved and "jump in."

Decentering should therefore be experienced in a stimulating atmosphere, without undue fear of not being able to do it, but with curious enthusiasm for doing it. Only in this way can the original problem in the client's concern fade into the background for this time. Usually, the atmosphere becomes optimal when the client and facilitator come into an aesthetic resonance.

This means that they also allow expressions about the emerging work that come from the sensorial: being touched, excited, moved, tense, etc. We speak in this context of the aesthetic responsibility of the therapist or counselor. We understand this as the responsibility of the professional facilitator towards the emerging work. It determines the interventions that enable the client to meet the artistic challenge with the resources available.

The artistic activities within our decenterings, motivated by exploratory curiosity while keeping everyone's cultural interest alive, can develop in this way from "art brut," "minimal music," everyday poetry, "poor theater" (Grotowski, 1968), collage techniques, and forms of contemporary performance art or installation art. Sometimes they also approach folk art, folk music, singing traditions, rap, freestyle jazz, or Western fusions of ethnic music, drum, or dance forms. However, there should always be a comprehensible relationship to it for all participants, even if it is only a curiosity to "get up close and personal with this something."

The understanding of aesthetics behind this didactic is culturally "polyphonic" and contradicts a simplistic distinction between "high" and "low" art. It is also an aesthetic that embraces the wide range of forms and styles accessible to us through cultural anthropology. Stige (2001) calls this aesthetic understanding "carnivalistic." It allows for combinations that include the tragic, the sublime, and the vulgar. Such an understanding, despite its multiple aspects, is clearly related to the senses. In our understanding, aesthetics is the logic of the senses; it is through the senses that meaning is to be experienced, witnessed, and perceived.

We derive the term aesthetics from the Greek stem: *aisthesis*. It is translated from ancient Greek as breath, from modern Greek as "through the senses." In the linguistic expression of an aesthetic experience, references to the corresponding senses become recognizable—"I am touched," "I am moved"—and in relation to breath, "It is breathtaking."

This understanding of aesthetics is the basis for structure and process in decentering and leaves a wide scope for client motivation. We call the resulting method "low-skill–high-sensitivity."

Low-skill–high-sensitivity

In different cultures, there are different design concepts and materials that lead to forms that are unfamiliar to us. Nevertheless, they often touch us precisely in their simplicity. In Western culture, some have learned that the quality of art lies in the perfection of manual dexterity, which allows the material to be perfectly structured to form in time and space. If we take a closer look, and especially if we consider the cultures of other parts of the world, we can see again and again that it is not always the virtuosity of the hand that makes the mastery of the work, but often a sensitivity towards the material of design and its qualities.

For example, we are enthralled by the perfect arithmetic traces around stones matched in size, shape, and texture in a Zen garden, or by flowers arranged in the Japanese style, even though the craftsmanship is secondary to the sense of color, shape, texture, and malleability of the material. Similarly, we are impressed by the extraordinarily purposefully juxtaposed ametric rhythmic sounds and noises punctuated by silence in exquisite timbres and dynamics of a Japanese Kabuki orchestra.

The expertise required for this lies in the ability to distinguish and employ these sound and noise qualities and structural contrasts. This expertise, in turn, is different from the kind of virtuosity we know from a classical violinist. The same is true of the dances and simple melodies of Native Americans, developed from their walking step and pulse. They shape the forward, backward, sideways, and "in place" in a choreography that refers to the architecture of the village square and its geometry in the form of a moving crystal.

It is a beauty that allows this form of dance to exist alongside the "acrobatics" of classical dance. The simple theater, as used by the Senoi to improvise dreams (Jennings, 1995), and the haiku tradition, a form of folk poetry in Japan, are other examples of the riches of low-skill–high-sensitivity design. In summary, one could say, analogous to craft training, these forms of design train the senses in a competent manner (Knill *et al.*, 1993).

With this representation from other cultures, it is by no means meant to say that we should imitate these traditions when decentering. Moreover, it should be noted that other traditions of artistic creation with very high standards of craftsmanship and virtuosity also exist in the above-mentioned cultures (Indian classical music, Chinese opera, polyrhythmic drumming in Africa, and many others). For its part, the low-skill–high-sensitivity concept is a very influential design principle in the contemporary art scene, "art brut," and folk art. Those mentioned above—"minimal music," installation art, performance art, collages, etc.— also belong to it.

It would be a misunderstanding if, with this way of looking at things, one of the two directions of art creation were to be given more value. We find both side by side in art, music, and the theatrical world today. What is essential in our context is that this principle, which places sensory competence before trained craft, has a tradition in all cultures and is very well suited to approaching a play or artistic work that allows for an aesthetic experience that is, again, not outside of our cultural involvement and outside of what we might call beautiful or appealing.

In conclusion, the principle of low-skill–high-sensitivity in the counseling or therapy situation captures, among other things, the quality and aspiration focus of creative and artistic work in order to motivate people who are distant from design or play-inhibited to decenter. As a rule, low-threshold and at the same time aesthetically appealing impulses are given. "Low skill" emphasizes the deliberate avoidance of technically demanding tasks and procedures. In contrast, there is a high degree of sensitivity concerning the handling of form, color, material, movement, time, space, expression, etc., and with regard to the detailed and careful reflection of the design process

Steps to raise sensitivity and motivation

Once the counselor has decided to engage in a particular play- or art-oriented process, the client should be made aware of the design elements step by step. For our methodology, we have divided the design elements into categories:

- **spatial and temporal framework** (canvas, stage, length of improvisation, etc.)
- **material sources** (various musical instruments, painting utensils, props, etc.)
- **material and/or structural properties** (color qualities, timbres, texture, etc.)
- **tools** (painting tools, drumsticks, stage lights, etc.)
- **design latitude** (setting limits—e.g., stepping out of the walk into the dance, modeling blindly, choosing only two colors, using two props).

As we will show later in Table 4.2, these categories are of different manifestations in each play or art discipline. The goal of a careful introduction, guidance, and completion of the decentering process is to involve the client with all his senses and to make him curious. Allowing the event to degenerate into casualness should be avoided, even if some of the elements may be trivial in another context. We think, for example, of the use of everyday objects in an installation structure, the use of sounds in a voice improvisation, newsprint in a mobile, or stones in a throwing game.

This usually results in the following series of steps (although the examples show that the sequence varies depending on the situation and takes place with smooth transitions):

- **Stake out and explore the framework.** The design space (stage, studio, screen, etc.) with its possibilities should be made familiar, and the timing clarified.
- **Attuning the senses involved** (e.g., before sculpting/modeling, the hands can be warmed by rubbing them together, then the warmth of the hands can be felt at a small distance from the cheek, etc.).
- **Exploratory selection.** The design materials and tools that are optionally provided require exploration and sensory exploration (physical warm-up, meditative attention, etc.).

For dance, this includes warm-up, stretching, and sensorimotor awareness. In music, it is the choice of a musical instrument. In design, it is the selection of pictures for a collage.

- **Experimenting with the design.** The design suggestions should avoid routine. This can be achieved by letting the participants try out unusual things (modeling blindfolded for a certain time, needing a fantasy language on stage, playing the strings instead of the keys on the piano, etc.). It also helps if the sensory perception is enriched by an unusual perspective (when creating, pay attention to the space between oneself and the dance partner instead of the body itself; physically feel the "dancing" movement when painting; listen to what the other players are playing on their instruments while you play yourself, etc.).
- **Making the emerging work perceptible as a partner in the process.** In the accompaniment, the circularity between leading and following, in the encounter with the work, should be sensitized again and again. Following the work becomes conscious by enriching the perception (intermediate feedback) and by asking questions that emphasize the "dance between the creator and the created" (e.g., "Let the piece lead you!" "How does the piece lead?" "With which form, which color, which rhythm does it lead?" "Where does the piece lead?" "What else does it need?").

The engagement, on the other hand, can be intensified if we encourage trial and error and emphasize the continuation in the work process by the creator. It helps if we refer to the tradition of "courageous" trial and error in the arts and in play. We then invoke the courage that creators of art need to overcome the inhibition that stands at every beginning. For example, before the risky intervention with the brush in the emptiness of the white canvas, with the first sound that falls in the silence, or during the process before each next act, whether in dance, theater, on the canvas, or in writing on paper. Whether this rehearsing "works out" or not is always revealed in hindsight. If we don't try anything or don't follow the process, nothing will be formed. What remains important is the intensive being-with-the-senses in the perception of what is happening and the friendly, open attitude towards surprises.

This series of steps can be captured using the acronym SERA as a thought guide. It gives keywords to the steps that should follow staking out the framework in smooth transitions:

- **S** for sensitization, in the exploration of the framework and in the attunement
- **E** for explorative and discovering selection
- **R** for the repetitive and circular in trying out
- **A** for the appreciation of the emerging work.

Not all steps can, of course, take up the same amount of time in each session. It is necessary to take into account in the current session the learning effect in terms of the play- and art-oriented design of previous sessions. There are also situations where a whole decentering is determined by one or two of these steps. Here is an example.

A team (in a team development assignment) agrees to do a dance improvisation in decentering. The coach uses all the available time for the dance ensemble's space and body awareness on the theme of closeness and distance during this first time where dancing takes place. The theme is first explored between dancers and studio boundaries, and then as closeness and distance between the dancers themselves. Of course, relatively close to the theme of the team—movement space, closeness, distance—this results in a rich harvest, even without taking further steps to create the work. This learning experience of the team as a dance ensemble can be built upon in the next dance improvisation.

To get an idea of what decentering looks like, involving all the steps, two progressions are shown here in outline style.

A music improvisation (concrete music) in an individual coaching session

Attunement: Time awareness as a frame, actually the second step, often comes within the first step in music. With blindfolded or (closed eyes), pay attention to the ambient sounds, then to what is sounding from within, both in silence. Then notice what noises, sounds, tones disturb, what pleases, and what sounds create a longing.

Exploratory choosing: Selecting from among the available sound sources (possibly musical instruments) that can produce sounds, noises that please. It can be a strange, a longing, or even a disturbing sound, but not something that leaves one indifferent.

Trying out designing: Using the selected instruments or sound-generating objects, try out different motifs (small sound sculptures). They do not have to have a metric pulse (beat). The experimentation takes 2–3 minutes. At least two motifs should be chosen. There should also be deliberate "silences" or pauses between the sounds or noises.

Making the emerging work perceptible as a partner in the process: An improvisation with the chosen motifs of 3–5 minutes should attempt to create a musical flow from the relationship of the motifs, a kind of sound tapestry. The improvisation is repeated, with brief feedback in-between, until a satisfying tapestry of sound emerges.

A shoe installation with a team in a supervision session

Attunement: In a meditative way, reflect on what you are wearing on your skin at the moment—how it feels, where it pinches, etc. Look at each other without speaking. Later, focus on the feet, becoming aware of what kind of shoes we wear in different situations, are wearing now, and how we feel in them.

Stake out and explore the framework: Clear out part of the workspace and mark it as an exhibition space for a collective installation with shoes, as might happen in a gallery (examples might include Beuys or Tinguely). Step back a bit from this space and see from different perspectives if the size and light allow. Then maybe put something (chair or table or bicycle) in it in a "denatured" position.

Exploratory selection: Leave the room to explore again on one's own what on the feet holds now the most attention (shoe, slipper, or sock). Re-enter the room with the choice made in the hand and the heightened awareness of the history of this object and personal attraction or rejection.

Trying out designing: With the object now in the hand and not on the foot and the gaze possibly on the sole and not on the upper, individually, without speaking, create unfamiliar encounters. Giving the shoe or sock its independence by setting it up differently and encountering it as an object still life as if a photographer. It is important to find surprising and interesting images.

Making the emerging work perceptible as a partner in the process: Now, the team assembles the shoes in the exhibition framework in various attempts to create a collective installation.

First exploration: Participants move only their own objects until silence occurs.

Second exploration: All objects can be moved by everyone; only one's own may not be moved ("Observe what your shoe or sock can also do when it becomes independent; you may take it in your hand again later if it is necessary").

Third exploration: The final movements involve only one's own object, and only if it is absolutely necessary.

Steps to enhance an inspiring studio atmosphere

Sometimes the studio or atelier mood is further enhanced when there is an aesthetic response from the therapist or counselor—that is, when the client receives feedback in an artistic form (a poem in response to an installation or a sound sculpture in response to a dance, etc.). Above all, this possibility is suitable within the situation where the client is creating and the person guiding is in the observational role.

Please note:

- Counselors may become too absorbed in their own activities and miss important observations or interventions.

- Explanatory interpretations may be hidden in the aesthetic response that misses the spirit of decentering.

An aesthetic response, on the other hand, is helpful in situations where the counselor's observational role triggers stressful performance pressures or expectations of getting graded due to proximity to a classroom situation. With media that offer participation, the counselor can take on the accompanying role in such situations. For example, the counselor may contribute musical improvisation to the dance ensemble. It is also possible to provide stage, lighting, and prop consultation and responsibility in theatrical improvisation.

In many activities, such as painting, designing, or writing, the studio atmosphere can become more natural if the counselor is also busy doing creative work, for instance.

It should be kept in mind that in all these activities, attention is focused on the process in a way that provides guidance responsibility.

Most of these decenterings are longer episodes lasting half an hour or more. There is often not enough time for this in the work with individual clients. The session with Hortense, described in detail above, and other examples described in this book show how something like a studio atmosphere can be created even in short decentering phases of five, ten, or fifteen minutes. The posture (including body posture) of the professional plays an important role. Even if she does not actively participate, it is important that she is present both outwardly and inwardly.

Our practical experience shows that the manner of instruction can contribute to an inspiring studio atmosphere and enhance motivation. It helps to:

- be interested in this way of creating and in the artistic media used
- choose a stimulating way of instruction
- react to impulses from clients, from the group, or from the team
- emphasize the experimental character and make the process transparent. Clients need to know what they are consenting to.

Instructions for explorations and their choice of possibilities should have an enticing, appropriate scope. Multiple offers can be stifling, and too much restriction can lead to blocking and boredom. Jean Piaget's reflections on intelligence development in the section on "Less is more" below help somewhat here (Knill *et al.*, 2004). We have coined the guiding principle "Less is more" from this for our practice.

"LESS IS MORE"—A GUIDING PRINCIPLE FOR INSTRUCTIONS REGARDING PLAY OR ARTISTIC CREATION

Jean Piaget's theory explains that differentiation of new patterns (related to action and/or intelligence) occurs in a process of accommodation and assimilation through playful exploration rather than "pattern transfer." This exploratory differentiation is motivated by curiosity and has a developmental direction from the rather diffuse to the more and more differentiated. For the motivation, it is important to grant an optimal playing field that allows this differentiation of new patterns. If it is too limited, only familiar, limited patterns are actually possible, the chances for discoveries are minimal, and the challenge remains uninteresting. If, on the other hand, the playing field is too wide, the situation can be so overwhelming that the client gives up or seeks refuge in old patterns.

The instructions for a design or play area in a decentering must therefore carefully consider several factors:

- the client's abilities
- the cultural background of the client
- the client's previous experience with such procedures and processes
- the available design materials and the equipment of the practice space.

The guiding principle "less is more" helps in providing instructions. It builds on the experience that the "less" of the play or design field, as well as the framework and material sources, allow for more discoveries and differentiations than a "more." However, it has also been shown that more than one direction needs to be offered for exploratory selection and experimental design in order to maintain a client's curiosity.

MORE is also an acronym that summarizes the rules that set the framework:

- **M**aterial: accessible to the client, (somewhat) familiar to the counselor (source material, tools, etc.)
- **O**rganization: simple rather than complex, but unfamiliar directions of exploration
- **R**oom and time: limited rather than spread out (framework)
- **E**xclusions and constraints: simple rather than complex.

For example, limiting the setting to one paper size, the source material exclusively to watercolor, or the choice of material only to two colors can inspire a great curiosity for discovery and allow freedom as the design style and use of water are taken in unfamiliar directions.

Interestingly, the guiding principle of "less is more" also warns against excessive or exclusive attention to creative exploration in differentiating new design patterns. While differentiation of new patterns emerges through exploratory play and is motivated by curiosity, mastery of the newly acquired occurs through repetition. The associated motivational force is captured by Karl Bühler's pedagogical term "*Funktionslust*" (the pleasure of being able to do it) (Mogel, 1990, p.23). This desire to repeat what succeeds must also be given space; this can mean that we pause without further exploration stimuli or additional specifications and simply repeat something with the stimulus of sensually perceiving it more completely.

The play or artistic process thus draws its fascination from three sources:

- exploring out of curiosity, which brings new forms and shapes into appearance
- repeating out of the pleasure of being able to do it in order to grasp and master the new
- letting oneself be challenged out of joy to prove oneself.

All three of these modes are of great importance, and each has a different character in the various arts. Thus, "ephemeral" creations, such as the performing or performative arts (music, dance, theater, performance, and all free plays), by their very nature, live as a result of repetition. They are temporal and can only be perceived in the repeated performance. Designs with materializable works and objects, on the other hand, such as the visual arts, are also perceptible without repetition.

There is often a reluctance on the part of professionals to use ephemeral means in decentering. Related to this is the sense of helplessness in the face of repetition, which is a prerequisite for being able to grasp the progress of the process. The request to repeat an improvisational work (theater scene, rap, jazz dance chorus, etc.) evokes negative memories of "rigid rehearsals" and negative experiences with rehearsals in which memorization and indoctrinating copying of formal aesthetic patterns were in the foreground.

The following section presents a work-based didactics that facilitates instruction in decentering with performing arts and with free play. This didactics derives from the experience with the tradition of improvisationally elaborated works, such as in jazz, blues, impromptu theater, performance, storytelling, and dance theater. This tradition understands "rehearsal" as an ongoing process of creation that continues until a meaningful form arrives. A form that emerges in this way can also be taken up again but remains alive in such a way that it is probably recognizable as a work (such as "Take Five" by Brubeck) and yet is also shaped by the moment each time. This principle is especially true in play-oriented decentering, where the repetition of play out of the pleasure derived from functioning brings forth new elements of mastering a creative process that later become important in aesthetic analysis and harvesting.

DIDACTICS RELATED TO THE WORK

We refer to work-related didactics as the way in which work-oriented decentering is instructed. It provides guidance on how to make the best use of the design possibilities of the work process.

Actually, work-related didactics is a condition of any work-oriented decentering. It emphasizes that a creative process is inconceivable without the work, even if it remains unfinished. If a painting has not been "finished," we are nevertheless faced with a canvas that is not empty, a "work in process." Process and work are obviously interdependent in any artistic creation, but play and playing are also interdependent in the broadest sense. After a free play in a decentering, I can always ask: "And what kind of game was that?" or "What was the name of the game?" or "What was decisive in the game finally working or becoming exciting?"

Work-related didactics also places an important emphasis on decentering as a method. After all, when we master a composition (even if the work is not yet complete), we have a sensory sense of accomplishment in a situation that challenges through constraint. This is opposed to the original feeling of inability in the situational limitation of the *Notenge*. Out of "aesthetic obligation" to the emerging work, the counselor empowers the client to take on the artistic challenge with the resources at his disposal, thus bringing the work to completion.

In the case of the visual arts and writing, it is more natural to speak of the "piece," since what is designed—the drawing, the poem, the sculpture, the short story, the installation, or other—can be viewed independently of the designer and the time, and without necessarily requiring any further design contribution. Therefore, it is not surprising that many directions of artistic therapies using these material means have always included the created object and the process in their method (McNiff, 1988).

This is much less the case with the forms of therapy that work with dance, music, or theater. The process comes to the foreground in these forms, also because a process is set in motion for each performance. However, it was soon understood that, for this reason, dance, music, performance, or theater also have the character of a piece of work. These types of creations (songs, dances, stories, theater, ritual games, etc.) also belong to all cultures.

ESSENTIAL ASPECTS OF WORK-RELATED DIDACTICS

For the time being, we must remember that traditional folk music, rock and pop music, jazz, folk dance, storytelling, slapstick, etc., are mostly improvisational. That is, first, they were not written down to begin with, and, second, they are interpreted anew, often substantially differently, each time out of the moment. Today, it is also postmodernism that performs improvisational works as performance works. These works are then also given names by which we have come to know them—for example, in the Living Theatre ("Paradise Now"). These improvisational paths to the work resemble making oneself familiar with a person.

Every encounter reveals new sides, perhaps also some that surprise in some way. Sometimes I discover so much that is different that I wonder if it is the same person. And yet, when I think about the next appointment, I will be aware that I have made an appointment with this person and no other. If I am friends with this person without being biased, then for me there is an identity between the (unchanging) name and the person, and yet the relationship remains alive and allows for change.

This state illustrates as a metaphor the completion of the improvisational work. Now, in the tradition of this kind of work elaboration, there is a classical form, which we call impromptu playing. It refers to the way of improvising, for example, a natural yodel, a 12-bar blues, or a *Schnitzelbank*. In impromptu playing, the laws of interplay are closely tied to a style. For our purposes, these sources are well suited if one can build on some experience with the client, and that is not at all uncommon when one becomes familiar with the folk material. We discuss below the essential aspects that apply to all forms (classical as well as modern).

The most important frame aspect in improvisation is *time*. Indeed, space has a fundamental importance, especially in dance, theater, play, and performance art. However, in any improvisation, we are also in a kind of time window that opens to imaginary reality and transforms space and time. Therefore, no instructions should be given during this time. Those who have instructed mainly painting, modeling, or writing, where the language of instruction can be adequate to the process, must become very accustomed to the fact that instructions are tremendously disturbing in an improvisation that itself includes sound and language. For this reason, all indications necessary for an improvisation must be announced before a time window is opened. In particular, attention should be given to the duration and how the end is indicated. We call these time windows "takes" (take one, take two, etc.) in the studio tradition.

Verbal announcements about the approaching end of a take (e.g., "It's time to stop") are perceived as disturbing within the imaginary reality of the play. Here, too, the "magic" of the studio is suitable—depending on the genre, a bell, light signal, "cut," hand signals, etc. The beginning of a take should also demand this kind of tension of silence and concentration, and this can be achieved with the same or similar signals. If we take into account, first, that more than one take is helpful in a session to capture changes, and second, that there must be time for studio reflection between takes, and third, that what has been created wants to be captured in the further process, then the optimal time for a take, as we will show later, is 3–4 minutes.

The instructions before a take should, in principle, consider all the design elements and motivational steps as presented in the "low-skill–high-sensitivity" practice. The "less is more" principle is particularly applicable. Keeping in mind that too much information tends to inhibit an improvisation and will be immediately forgotten anyway, it is recommended to include a preparatory phase, which can be verbally accompanied, before introducing the improvisation model. After the framework has been explored in this sensorial attunement and the direction of exploration of the design material has been initiated, the improvisation model can be introduced or developed with the client. The following examples will illustrate this.

In a sensitivity-raising introduction to a dance improvisation, warming up the body can be achieved, for example, through breathing and stretching exercises on all levels (standing, on all fours, and on the floor) with a simultaneous awareness of the different perspectives. The instruction that follows will invite exploration of the studio space as a frame as the dancers move through these three planes. As a design exploration, each dancer can now try out a level and dance style and make a choice. All this can be accompanied by verbal observations and commented on at any time for motivation.

Now the improvisation model can be developed with the clients from the explored elements. The characteristics of the movements, the dancers and their levels, and the choice of music and rhythm could be discussed. Then the first take is done as an experiment, without any verbal guidance.

It looks similar in a play activity. To warm up, the client explores all the game objects provided (stones, screws, pieces of wood, marbles, etc.), touches and "grasps" them, weighs them up, and tries out what is possible with them. Then he prepares and explores the framework of the playing field, and, finally, he chooses the material and the way of playing. The consultant can accompany all this verbally and observationally; she can also intervene and motivate.

Now comes the first attempt at play, which, like a take in improvisation, without interrupting commentary by the counselor, should allow the client to immerse himself completely in the play for a time.

Practice shows us repeatedly that it is effective to start with a brief first draft of an improvisation model or playing approach. The time for the first take or playing phase should also be rather short (2–3 minutes). It helps to point out that instead of trying to decide what is perfect by discussing it for a long time, we try it by acting first and then make changes out of experience before the second take. This attitude also lowers expectations that are too high. Time and again, moreover, in the discussions between takes or play approaches, attention must be drawn to the fact that more attempts will follow and that we will make decisions out of action. If the work or play is then "on the way" or "gets it right," the time can be extended, but usually a time has already settled in beforehand that no longer requires an end mark.

Each take needs a debriefing that leads into the preliminary discussion of the next take. It should also be short because play and creation have priority during decentering. The following guide lists the points that can be touched upon in such an intermediate discussion. The emphasis should be different in each conversation. It is not advisable to cover all the main points in detail each time, but it is useful to explore all the possibilities in the course of decentering, for example.

Feedback from the creator(s) about the improvisation and/or feedback from the witnesses by the director or any teammates

Feedback questions: "What works?" "What surprises?" "What is the biggest challenge?" etc.

Ask for wishes about what else could happen or be tried: "What would you like to change? Is there anything new coming?"

After the second and subsequent takes or play approaches, "Is it on track?" "Is anything showing yet?" "What does it take to get on track?" "What could be left out or picked up again?" "How far along are you with the play?" "Is the work noticeable now?" "How do you notice it?" "What helped?" "What was getting in the way last time?" "How did you overcome it?" etc.

Do we need a change in the improvisation model or game approach, or should we just try it again? Changes can be suggested by the client or facilitator.

Instructions and feedback must be as concrete as possible. They must remain on the surface, so to speak. This applies not only later in the aesthetic analysis but also here in the interim discussions, between takes and playing approaches. When and where something happened in an improvisation is important, but so is what exactly happened when. How could it have been seen or heard? No feedback should begin without the addressee confirming that they know exactly what it refers to. The language should remain with the studio language. Accurate designations from the design element categories help.

Those who predominantly have experience in instructing the visual arts are used to the fact that the framework—for example, through the size of the paper—is almost a given. In general, many of these details hardly need to be mentioned in the fixed design media and their design elements, since they are implicitly already prepared that way. This applies, among other things, to the general conditions, the paper format, the choice of source material, the oil pastels, and the time, which can be continuously directed verbally. The counselor will have to get used to the fact that in the performing arts, the indications about the time frame, the material sources, tools, or the exploration direction have to be mentioned very precisely, concretely, and explicitly at the beginning and in the intermediate discussions.

Before a second take, the client will often remark that he is no longer able to create the same improvisation. Here the comparison we used above in connection with Living Theatre helps—namely, to compare the improvisational path to the work with becoming acquainted with a person. In our context here, meeting and making friends with a new acquaintance will awaken the understanding that it is about one and the same process of discovery and that there are surprises. Also, the comparison with painting can clarify that it is always about the same canvas when we work on a composition; and there too, especially at the beginning of the painting process, the image will change amazingly from visit to visit, and only from a certain point onwards will the work emerge clearly.

THE DESIGN ELEMENTS AND THEIR FEATURES

As we have shown, the motivation to engage in creating depends on the instructor's ability to introduce the design elements in a way that makes them sensory and appealing. Instructions are more effective if we have an appropriate vocabulary for each design element. To assist instructors, we have developed a table based on the categories introduced in the low-skill–high-sensitivity section (framework, material sources, material and/or structural properties, tools, and design scope).

The schematic representation tries to exemplify the terms for some selected disciplines of artistic creation. The representation is far from being a definition in the tradition of formal aesthetics or from making a claim to completeness. However, with the examples listed, it aims to give counselors and therapists a basis for grasping the design elements to develop the vocabulary in the instructions themselves.

We will see that the variety of distinctions depends in each case on the art discipline and its stylistic expression. In music, for example, the choice of material source, musical instrument, sound object, or one's voice is of utmost importance and requires attention and time. In dance, on the other hand, there is no choice of the tool; there is no other tool than the dancer's physical body, which shapes space through movement. Attuning the body as a tool is of great importance here.

The distinction in the category of frames is differently determining in different art traditions. They are mainly defined by the tradition in the arts. But it is equally a tradition of the arts to break the frame with a new discipline, which then leads to a new style. The frame condition "unity of time, space, and action" in theater and its continuity was broken by cinema. With the "flashback," film also introduced a new stylistic element for literature. The tradition that provided for a two-dimensional frame in painting (the drawing, the engraving, etc.) was broken by contemporary painters who paste three-dimensional objects into the picture with paint or glue. These and other examples show that this kind of disciplined frame-breaking always means more imagination and not necessarily more craftsmanship. For decentering in the "low-skill–high-sensitivity" style, the adoption of such or similar stylistic elements is therefore very suitable.

For example, a performance improvisation could be moved up and down the stairwell instead of on a fixed stage. A sculpture could be mounted on wheels and equipped with wind sails. Choreography is created by the actors puffing.

Table 4.2 Distinguishing features in the comparison of art disciplines

Example differentiation possibilities

Types and styles of art	Frame: spatial, temporal	Sources of material
Visual arts: Painting, drawing, digital photography, or image work	Canvas, paper, cardboard, plywood, etc., and their size	Watercolor, acrylic, colored pencils, wax crayons, charcoal, finger paint, etc. A digital camera, computer
Installations	Stage-like setting, mark size	Already formed objects from nature, found objects, personal items (clothes, jewelry, etc.)
Woodcarving	The "inner space" in the selected block	Tree trunks, logs, etc., and their character, shape, and size
Music: action music, e.g., Kabuki music	Formed in a space of time, so to speak, into silence Duration	Musical instruments or objects that "resound"
Free vocal improvisation	Formed in a space of time, so to speak, into silence Duration	The human voice, female/male voices, speaking/singing voice, etc.
Traditional forms (folk songs, rap, blues, etc.).	Formed in a space of time, so to speak, into silence Duration	Human voices or musical instruments

Dance	Studio or stage, three-dimensional space and time	Space and movement, objects (e.g., chairs, ball), if they are fixed in space as architecture
Verse, poetry, word improvisation	Writing room, reading stage, "writing screen," etc.	Language elements, dialect, letters, consonants, vowels, syllables, words
Theater: The poor theater	Stage space and time	Situation, scene, script
Puppetry	Puppet stage and time	Puppets, stories, and scenes, etc.

Differentiation possibilities

Material and/ or structural properties	Tools	Scope for design
Colors, texture, shapes, lines, brushstrokes, etc.	Brushes, knives, rollers, spatulas, etc., and their properties: wide, narrow, soft, pointed, hard, etc.	Start with eyes closed or with movement of hands, follow what catches your eye, etc.; free, abstract, non-representational, representational, etc.
Spatial references, degree of unfamiliarity, etc.: near, far, connected, separate, etc.	Hands or tools, etc.	Place objects in sensitive perspective of the whole: stacking, arranging, serializing, etc.
Woodgrain, grown and formed structures, hardness, color, etc.	Knife, chisel, hammer, saw, axe, etc.; the cutting-edge characteristics, etc.	Carving with the grain, following what has grown, etc.
Sound characteristics; timbre, pitch, length, volume, articulation, etc.	Hands, drumsticks, bows, brushes; heavy, light, soft, hard, etc.	Number of instruments, interplay, density, motifs, characters, development, spinning on, etc.
Sounds, tones, consonants, vowels, etc.; timbre, pitch, length, volume, articulation, etc.	The body of the musician, the vocal organ, the breath, etc.; standing or sitting, sotto voce, whispering, etc.	Metrical or ametrical rhythm, tempo, motives, figures, development, etc.; voice relationship: unison, harmony, contrapuntal, dissonant, etc.

Tones or speaking voice, timbre, pitch, length, volume, etc.	Vocal organ, breath/ hands, drumsticks, bows, articulation, text phrasing, etc.	Single or multiple voice rules, voice hierarchy, traditional patterns such as 12-bar or simple blues, etc.
Shaped space, "effort and shape," force flow, shaping mode, direction of motion, energy, etc.	The body of the dancers, ball, sticks, pillows (if actively involved in the movement)	Choreographic indications, the manner of the designed patterns
Everyday language; metaphorical, symbolic, reflexive, concrete, neological, etc.	Voice, pen, pens, pastels, paper size/ shape; computer; right or left hand	Free writing with the sound of language, giving voice to objects (persona or animate), collecting words, researching, etc.; forms such as haiku, sonnet, etc.
Action, roles, characteristics of roles, props, set design	Body, voice, speech, movement, etc.	"Plot," theme, action, improvisational structure, character and story development, etc.
Plots, puppet characters, props, scenery	Hands and voice	"Plot," theme, action, improvisational structure, character and story development, etc.

The above terms should not be taken as a starting point for work-oriented guidance of decentering. The counselor must first consider what kind of work he wants to address. Then the above distinctions can help to make the guidance concrete and the subsequent aesthetic analysis differentiated. Therefore, the division must not be taken literally. Sometimes a design material is more a source of material, and sometimes it can be understood more as a tool. If we paint with oil pastels, for example, we will differentiate them as a tool or as a source of material, depending on the design task. If the technique of rubbing the oil chalk is proposed, then the chalk is rather thr source of material, and the fingers are the tool, so to speak, brush. Without rubbing or scratching techniques, all chalks are both a source of material and a tool. Of course, there are combinations.

In a vocal improvisation with spoken language, speech could be offered as a source of material for the exploration of structural properties such as vowel sounds and consonant sounds, which can then be shaped according to the properties of timbre, duration, and volume. Alternatively, the human voice can be taken as a source of material, and the structural properties from singing voice to speaking voice can be proposed as differentiation of sounds and noises to an improvisation with long and short sound events. In both cases, the concept of tool is not in the foreground. We know compositions of this kind by Dieter Schnebel (1930).

Theme-near and theme-far decentering

In the course of our discussion, we have repeatedly illustrated how decentering by moving away from the problem—that is, away from the client's concern—in an alternative context allows for experiences that are conducive to resolution.

The problem identified in the interview from the client's concern usually involves different domains. It is then quite possible that one of the areas of concern emerges consciously or unconsciously in decentering without addressing the problem itself. For example, we might ask to what extent the issue of "communication" raised in a leadership problem can be brought into a theater. In this case, the decentering proceeds more or less obviously from the client's concern. This is understood as near-theme decentering.

In principle, it can be assumed that a theme related to the problem may appear as an explicit element even in the case of a well-achieved decentering. However, the essence of decentering is to shift the focus of attention to something other than the problem. The issues inherent in the problem are in the background in the alternative world experience. The same should be true for the counselor and therapist. It is contrary to the principle of decentering if the guidance is chosen from the idea of the solution. The "jumping ahead" of the counselor should also decenter him in such a way that he, competent and present, can devote himself primarily to the challenge of guidance.

The first thing that can be stated is that an issue should never appear in the play or the design in such a way that it brings the client back into the helplessness of the *Notenge* or occupies the guide in such a way that he only thinks about the solution of the problem.

As a second aspect, when decentering is successful, we can often find that a theme is also present in the structure of a play or artistic creation in an unplanned way, without the problematic limiting the possibilities of action. An example will illustrate this.

> **COACHING IN CONNECTION WITH EXAM ANXIETY**
> A theater improvisation is spontaneously proposed as decentering. As a scene, there is an office table with a boss and a visitor. The client wants to play the boss. A job interview is chosen for the improvisation. In the various takes, the play turns more and more into some sort of a comedy, after the client as the boss hides behind feudal office furnishings, clearly taking a liking to arrogant interruptions with phone calls and rude cigarette smoking. The client does not become aware of the problem (examination fears) during the elaboration of this "tale," although the play thematically comes close to a change of perspective from the examinee's point of view.

Decenterings that do not incorporate the client's concern or care into the structure of the guidance, or do so only in an unplanned way, are what we call theme-far decenterings.

When an aspect of a topic is included in the decentering on the counselor's instructions, we call it a theme-near decentering. This can happen in two ways:

- aspects of the theme are taken into the decentering
- something from the structure of the theme is taken over.

Methods such as playful change of perspective, role play, guided imagination, creative constellation of a situation, or installation are often close to a topic in terms of content and can bring about surprising openings; they can therefore also be used as short sequences to clarify the concern at the beginning of the session.

Adopting the structure of an existing problem is meaningful only if it can be spontaneously recognized out of a topic in such a way that an art discipline immediately comes to the counselor's mind. To discover such similarity of structures, one can take into account viewpoints of intermodal theory. For example, the interpersonal structure of the concern may provide a clue to the arts discipline that most closely matches that interpersonal viewpoint. For example, a team with a concern involving communication between members addresses a similar interpersonal structure as a free jazz ensemble. A "low-skill–high-sensitivity" musical improvisation could be chosen here.

The way in which a concern manifests itself can also give clues as to the direction of exploration. Here the crystallization principle (Knill, 1990b) is helpful in the choice of the type of design. If a concern is characterized by confusion due to a situation that never comes to rest, the structural similarity of "movement as modality" can be used in dancing, modeling, or painting without taking the problem into the design. Dance itself is crystallized movement because movement is the substance of dance, without which it is unthinkable. In dance, movement is experienced first-hand and can be reflected upon from the experience. In modeling/plasticizing and painting, the image is in the foreground, but the movement can also be captured, but—and this is important—in painting, the movement can be perceived from a distance. This difference can be decisive for the decision regarding the type of creative activity.

There is also the possibility of beginning very theme-near and increasingly decentering into theme-far. This is possible if one first defamiliarizes a situation of concern into a play (e.g., by placing or moving objects, figures, or items) and then takes what appears as an image, movement, action, or sound as the starting point for an artistic design. For example, one poses a situation with stones of different colors, shapes, and sizes.

Instead of going for the solution here, you decenter further and let this structure be completed as an artistic mosaic by adding another material (e.g., colored sand). Such mixed forms can help to soften the "exotic" of a decentering somewhat.

4.7 Analysis and feedback in decentering

We must keep in mind that clients are awake, aware, and responsive in the encounter with the guide throughout the extraordinary context of the session, including during decentering. It is then obvious that the experience during the decentering, which has led to a substantial, visible, and/or audible result, must be looked at closely. This is especially so since this process involves the actions and struggles of the same person who has reached limits with challenges in the everyday context. Now the same person, first in conversation, in taking up the concern, and then again now, in the challenge of decentering, is in an awareness-generating process of accompaniment. This continuous awareness and responsiveness must be used here, at the end of the decentering in the studio, by working out the analysis, looking into it from the client's perspective. For this, the work is the surface of observation, from which process questions can also be answered.

This observation is representation, a kind of aesthetic protocol of the range of play gained from the play and the creative. This surface of the work can also be seen from the perspective of self-organizational theory, first of all as a field in which attractors for new perspectives, ideas, and ways of seeing and acting can arise. Core principles of self-organizational understanding are also applicable to the artistic process. The attracting dynamics within the self-organization to the artistic work can be seen as analogous to the dynamics of a change process. This must be communicable and comprehensible in language in the analysis in order to have an effect in the context of everyday life.

Such a contemplation also causes an ego-distancing. This means that the artistic-playful expression is, on the one hand, not conceivable without the acting creator and involves her bodily-emotionally, but that, on the other hand, the work now visible in the world as a cultural phenomenon opens up something new and different in each case and thus, depending on the culture, enables multiple perspectives and meanings. This aspect is also important in the analysis if we want to reflect from a systemic point of view (Knill, 2004).

If we consider all these aspects, we are amazed at the tremendous wealth of perceivable substance that presents itself at the conclusion of a decentering. It has been shown that, all too often, we lose a large part of the "data." This can happen if we do not proceed very carefully. Often, for example, we allow ourselves to be seduced by a striking foreground and push towards the harvest, unaware of the wealth of important experiences that could have been perceived by the client.

We noticed that already in the course of a decentering the client made observations about the difficult or successful ways of proceeding and expressions about the work. These were then later appreciated during the harvesting only because the counselor or an outside observer had been taking notes.

We sometimes have the impression that what is not captured in the analysis is "blown away" after leaving the studio space. For all these reasons, we have developed an acronym as a guide to help us capture the richness of the "surface" very close to the concrete. This is to avoid the "superficiality" of a hasty reduction to a single interpretation. Because we mean that very specifically always close to the sensual perception of the thing itself, as manifested by the work-like concrete result, we speak of the " aesthetic analysis". In the Greek root word *aisthesis*, the reference to the senses is given.

Here we would still like to warn against the rigid handling of the acronym presented in the following. It should be remembered that we intend to have a conversation. Usually, conversations in the presence of an artistic work begin quite naturally with a first spontaneous expression, usually in the form of a kind of congratulation: "I'm amazed at the intensity of these colors!" or "This text grabbed me from A to Z!" or "I don't even know where to begin. There were so many surprises in the improvisation. So, for example, the sudden drop in of the speaking voices, etc." or "Oh, that was quick, wasn't it? And from where should we look?," etc.

We advise accompanying persons to remain authentic and sensitive to not falling into patterns that evoke inhibiting memories from negative biographical artistic experiences.

The acronym OPER

We will see that the order of levels of analysis suggested by this guide is significant. For the time being, an abridged version follows here.

- **O (Obvious) stands for surface.** This means the actual material or phenomenological manifestation of the result. That which becomes visible with the design, audible with the music, readable with the written, audible and visible with the theater, etc., is the surface.
- **P stands for process.** All measures, courses of action, strategies adopted, interventions, assistance, etc., related to

progress, obstacles, successes, what is satisfactory or unsatisfactory, etc.

- **E stands for experiencing.** The way the process phases and events were experienced—for example, surprises and emotional components.
- **R (realign/rough direction) stands for indications of direction.** Questions and comments regarding further editing or completion of the work: "What else does the work need?" "Is it finished? "If not, how would I proceed?" "What does the work have to say to me?" "What do I like about it?" "What is significant?" "Do I want to give it a name?," etc.

Surface

This is the actual aesthetic protocol of the entire decentering. In the next steps, this can be used for the aesthetic analysis of the process, the experiences, and what indicates the direction by pointing out, relating, and referring.

It is important to start from the analysis of the created, so to speak, from all that can be seen and heard. This is the fundamental difference from the other phenomena of imagination. The representational, thing-like nature of artistic activity and play allows a simultaneous, direct access for the client and the facilitator. During the very process of making, what is created can be seen and heard, touched and felt. In intervening, we are not solely dependent on description or interpretation; we experience ourselves confronted with a verifiable surface to which direct reference can be made.

On this surface, the self-perception can be checked against the perception of others. Often the works are taken over by habitual prejudices of judgment. In the clarifying conversation of the aesthetic analysis related to the surface, it is here that the view of the unnoticed is opened, and blind spots become obvious. Such corrections of the perception towards the created and its effect on the environment are probably of the greatest importance. Only when what is substantially present, the work, has been comprehensively perceived should an extended reflection on the ways of proceeding and of behavior be approached. Otherwise, it easily happens that essential aspects in the process or experience of the client, which are connected with important manifestations in the work, are passed over because of blind spots or rigid patterns of perception of the counselor. For this reason, the analysis of the surface should be done at the beginning.

The procedure for the analysis of the surface

This object of analysis is sensorially perceptible in the manner described above for a few selected artistic design disciplines in the section "The design elements and their features." According to Table 4.2, the categories can be used to proceed. It should be noted that not all categories are equally important in every design medium. Material and structural properties are always of primary importance; the other elements are often negligible. Some examples will outline this.

Questions about material and/or structural properties:

- **When painting:** colors, texture, shapes, lines, etc.
- **In theater:** plot, roles, role characteristics, props, set design, etc.
- **In free music improvisation:** sound characteristics, their timing and how they occur in timbre, pitch, length, volume, rhythmic patterns, etc.
- **In dance:** utilization of space, type of shaping, direction of movement, flow of force (effort and shape), etc.
- **In writing:** type of language, everyday, metaphorical, symbolic, reflective, concrete, neological, poetically condensed language, etc.
- And so on with other means of design.

Questions about sources of material:

- **In music:** sound sources or instruments; in what way, when? etc.
- **In theater:** situation, scene, script, etc.
- And so on with other design approaches.

Questions about the scope of design:

- **In writing:** aspects of form, such as rhythm, verse, paragraphs, references, flashbacks, etc.
- **In music:** number of instruments, interplay, density, motifs, figures, development, continuation, etc.
- And so on with other design approaches.

Questions about the frame:

- **In theater:** stage space and time-action frame.
- **In writing:** frame of a short story, essay, comedy, mystery, etc.
- And so on with other design tools.

Questions about tools:

- **In theater:** voice and body use, use of language, movement, etc.
- **In music:** using mallets (soft, hard), bows, hands, brushes, etc.
- And so on with other means of design.

It is best to complete the perception of decentering when an open conversation arises in the analysis that does not consist only of questions from the facilitator and answers from the client. It is beneficial if counselors and therapists also share their observations. These should stick to surface criteria and avoid reductive or generalizing interpretations. The effectiveness of such interventions is then most likely to be achieved when the place, the time, and the basis of the manifestation are observed for all to see and in the attitude of aesthetic responsibility. This could then proceed like this:

Consultant: "Your second gong beat brought the dense, rather forte percussion interaction to a close, and then in the fade, the stringed instruments appeared in a carpet-like weave. Do you know where that was?"

Client A: "No, I just remember my beat within the percussion improvisation, but yes, there was a change; what was that like?"

Client B: "I looked up at you; you switched to the big soft mallet at that point."

Client A: "Yeah, now I'm getting something; was that when it got so quiet?"

Counselor: "Yes, everyone paused, and all you heard was the wonderful fading of the gong, then it went on, remember?"

Client C bursts in: "Now it's my turn! Did I think at the fading of the gong, this is the time for my string psaltery—that fits!"

Client A: "Now I remember where that was, about halfway through the improvisation, right? Yes, that's important because I hadn't expected such a musical effect for the whole ensemble when I switched to the soft mallet."

Process

The artistic or play-oriented challenge in decentering has not only brought about a detachment from problem thinking but in this detached atmosphere has also led to an artistic solution. Now that this result, called "work," has been completed in perception and appreciated in its beauty, the conditions that led to the aesthetic result must also be recorded. This analysis must be done in a resource-oriented manner. This implies that the first step of the analysis has been done in the spirit of appreciating the work, and now it can be determined what resources came into play. The process analysis should bring up:

- **What was helpful**, how the idea came about, and from whom it came (client or facilitator).
- **What turned out to be superfluous** and what function it had for moving forward. Did it become an aid to decision-making, or did it create an important detour?
- **What was an obstacle**, and what made the client continue anyway.

In this reflection, the following aspects are integrated:

- everything that was provided in terms of frameworks, material sources, and tools, or what clients additionally requested or did not use

- the design and play instruction of the process facilitator at the beginning and during the process
- all questions, suggestions, actions, and spontaneous, planned, and unplanned events from the client perspective during the process and in the improvisations between the "takes."

It is quite possible to equate this analysis with the mobilization of resilience. According to Schiffer, resilience is the ability to activate resources (Schiffer, 2001, p.11). Here in this analysis, situations are captured that have to do with choice and constraint, dealing with obstructive and helpful actions, spontaneity and accident, chance and planning, autonomy, and accepting help. Everything is reflected in terms of what has been achieved in the design and the play; it is shown how both "positives" and "negatives" become manageable for solutions.

This perspective also explains why this process analysis often produces sentences that sound like pearls of wisdom in their poetic quality. For example, a client who was at a loss when painting later answered the question in the process analysis as to what had finally brought her forward: "You simply have to take a few steps back, then you regain the bigger picture."

One client on the team directs a theater improvisation and remarks after the second take in the planning conversation for the third take, "If I don't have everyone performing at the same time, you can see the joke better, and it becomes humorous."

It is advisable to take notes during the process. For improvisations, this can be done on the flipchart in the form of stage directions. The sheet can then be filled in further during the analysis of the process.

Experiencing

Naturally, experiential content will already be incorporated within the surface and process analysis. In this phase of the aesthetic analysis, the experience should move to the center. It is advantageous to note the moments where signs of emotion or excitement were perceived earlier in the analysis conversation. Here we will now address them. There are two important reasons for dealing with experiential content earlier only in the case of intense emotional reactions:

- The perception of what has been achieved is only now completed. Before that, there is the danger of a perception limited by convictions. In the case of strong emotions about the work that has been created, it is helpful to briefly give these space so that perception is freed up for aesthetic analysis.
- The resources are now activated, and we can build on resilience.

The conversation at this stage focuses on events such as:

- "What was surprising?" "Where were you pleased, shocked, or annoyed?"
- "How was your state physically and psychologically before decentering and now in comparison?" "Did you notice anything about this state in between?"
- "How did you experience your co-participants—before, after, in-between?"
- "How did you experience our relationship during decentering?"

It is easy to be tempted to make references to the concern in the everyday context at this stage of the analysis, but we should wait until the harvest to do this. Otherwise, all the data collected beforehand may be hastily subsumed under this one aspect.

Particularly in this phase of the analysis, a resource-oriented attitude should be cultivated. In the case of positive experience contents, the question "What else?" should lead to further information. In the case of negative experience contents, the question about what helped to stay with it anyway is important. The request to the client to present what could have happened instead often has a place here as well.

Pointing in the direction

Here, at the end of the aesthetic analysis, the focus is on the work or the play as it is now visible in the world as a cultural phenomenon and in relation to the client's other works. Each work opens up something new and different in each case, allowing for multiple perspectives and meanings depending on the culture. Only in the following step, the harvesting, is the search for meaning in relation to the client's concern and everyday context. Here it is a matter of becoming aware that what has emerged in the decentering is *meaningful.*

We also remember "what is beyond our control," "what happens in dreams as in art." This surprising, even beautiful something deserves awe and appreciation. Room should also be given to a kind of gratitude.

The following topics can be addressed here:

- **The work, the improvisation, and its completion.** "What else is needed?" "How would you continue?" "Is there anything else that needs to be added?"
- **The work, the improvisation in conjunction with others.** "This improvised melody is in a folk minor key; it reminds me of an old love song!" "It reads like a mocking poem of the Basel Fasnacht!" "It's like the second act of the theater we performed two weeks ago!"
- **Does the work say something to me, does it speak to me?** "If it says something to you, what does it say?" "If it speaks to you, how does it speak?" "Does it have a title?"
- **Now, at the end of this review/work analysis**, what is particularly meaningful to you in the work? Symbolic aspects can also come up here. According to the phenomenological tradition, it is important to anchor all statements on the surface and keep them as open as possible.

Final remarks on the aesthetic analysis

Of course, the aesthetic analysis cannot always follow exactly this pattern of OPER. There is often a tendency for a very abstract level—for example, directional elements or interpretations of meanings—to be spontaneously introduced. It is not useful to stop so abruptly. On the other hand, it is helpful to lead the conversation back to the concrete surface whenever a leap forward into a more advanced level occurs and to anchor the conversation there.

So, for example, you can say, "Yes, and where does this become visible, here in the sculpture made of clay?" Or, "Was this when you went to the xylophone and developed the melody?" Then, when one is back at the surface, one can add to the perception from here and also address process questions that have to do with this addition. One then remarks, for example, "However, I also see in this sculpture this round protrusion next to the incision you mention; was that out of some other impulse?" Or, "Then you hummed the melody again later, on the monochord; were you aware that it was the same, a kind of reprise?"

OPER is intended as a guide to remind us, as we proceed in aesthetic analysis, to seek rich language as concretely as possible on the surface, and to be aware of it when we enter the realm of interpretation. For the harvest, where meanings are allowed to have room regarding the concern, having as rich a palette of "tangible" statements as possible is beneficial.

4.8 Yield for the everyday context—the "harvest"

The artistic or playful decentering, including its aesthetic analysis, is completed. Counselor and client are again seated on the chairs where the session began and the conversation about the concern and visions of the future took place. Thus, they have retaken their seats in the original conversation space and have returned, as it were, from the alternative to the extraordinary context of counseling.

The point now is to make the connection between what was initially discussed here and what happened during the decentering and its analysis. The starting point for this part of the conversation is an initial question formulated as openly as possible. Its purpose is to relate the experiences made during the decentering and the aesthetic analysis in all their diversity to what was discussed at the beginning of the counseling.

We refer to the search for possible relations between decentering events and the real situation as "harvesting." The term arose spontaneously. This term expresses that what can be harvested has something to do with the efforts of the client and the work of the professional but that the harvest cannot simply be produced. There is no procedure of any kind that determines the content of what is revealed in the harvest. It is not a matter of the most skillful associative or rational reasoning. What is harvested falls to the client, often comes as a surprise, and usually has the character of a (sudden) insight.

Open phrasing of the initial question

Of course, we would never claim to a client that there must be a certain connection/relationship here that needs to be figured out. We always speak of several connections and possible (i.e., hypothetical) relationships.

It is therefore counterproductive to first bundle the experiences during the decentering phase or to want to inquire about the "most meaningful" experience or even the essence of the experiences made. Through such efforts, the counselor would unduly narrow the search direction and suggest that there are important and unimportant or even "right" and "wrong" connections. On the contrary, it is by no means always the very first associations that prove fruitful and valuable in later processing.

Often, connections that emerge as "another possibility" only after some reflection are particularly stimulating and fruitful.

On the other hand, it is not only counterproductive but downright wrong to associate what has happened in the alternative context directly with the wording of the specific concern or even with the formulated "good outcome" of the current session. Previous experience shows that what can be "reaped" as a harvest almost always relates to something more fundamental, more general, and quite often has only an indirect connection to the wording of the concern formulated at the beginning of the session. It is therefore important to ask the question that introduces the conversational phase of harvesting very openly and to include both what is actually happening during the decentering and the aesthetic analysis.

The following examples indicate the type of formulation to think of.

"Now, looking back from here at the experience you had there, and everything that was talked about there [we're looking from our chairs to the place of decentering], what might that have to do with what you told me at the beginning of our conversation?"

"And now, if we relate everything that has happened and been discussed in the last 15 minutes to what came up at the beginning of the session, what comes to mind?"

"Suppose what happened over there [meaning in the play, the

> work, and the aesthetic analysis] had something to do with what we discussed at the beginning of the session, what might that be?"

Once this first question has been asked, the counselor must wait, simply wait, because the question is difficult. From the point of view of everyday logic, it is impossible, somehow "misplaced," since we expect an answer about a connection, where, for linear everyday thinking, there can be no connection at all. It is all the more astonishing that up to now all our clients have been able to answer this question without any assistance. Sometimes very quickly and spontaneously, sometimes only hesitantly and after a longer pause.

Assistance

A possibility to help is the simple repetition of the question asked, either verbatim or formulated as a variant. Assistance could also be to repeat the client's statement as literally as possible during the aesthetic analysis. In doing so, the counselor should avoid making personal additions or specifically emphasizing certain remarks made by the client. While it may be understandable that counselors who are not yet familiar with the procedure try to help the client, especially if they themselves see such possible connections, doing so at this point in the conversation is entirely contrary to the principal orientation of our way of working.

Only once in recent years have we received the answer "Nothing at all" (meaning: "I don't see any connection"). Spontaneously, the counselor responded something like this:

> Of course. After all, that's a completely absurd question. At the beginning of the session, you tell me about this difficulty in your institution. Then you work on this sculpture and do everything to make it as aesthetically beautiful as possible. And now I ask about the connection between the two. [Pause.] Suppose there were connections now, though. What kind could they be? I can reread what you said about your work and the process that led to it.

It did not come to that at all. The client interrupted the counselor and, without any urging on his part, was able to state a whole series of possible links. There was enough time to elaborate on two of them further. This made it possible to outline concrete ways of solving the problem. During a telephone conversation the following week, the client reported that she had used one of the options in the team meeting, which led to the first positive effects on the very same day.

The example shows that the first thing to do is to make associative connections between the alternative reality of decentering and the concerns and goal visions that the client has brought to the session—that is, between decentering events and the ordinary experience of the world.

Gather associations

At this point, it should be emphasized that it is beneficial to record all the connections that are assumed by the client as literally as possible. The emphasis is on the words "all" and on "record." First, we never leave it at a single hypothesized connection. And second, we write down the statements in order to be able to quote them as literally as possible at a later time, if necessary.

It is, therefore, not very helpful to ask for more detail on a single point or to allow the client to justify and detail an idea at great length. Other ideas, possibly those that are strikingly different from the associations expressed so far, might be lost. Only if a word or part of a sentence is not at all comprehensible is an inquiry appropriate. Everything else can be postponed for now. Any argumentation is counterproductive at this stage and also later! The best follow-up question is "What else?"

It is useful to ask this "What else?" question repeatedly. It pays off if different hypotheses are available. If this repeated "What else?" becomes slightly uncomfortable or even embarrassing to the asking counselor (rarely the client), one can switch to "Is there anything else?" or even to "Does another possible connection occur to you, or nothing more at the moment?"

Once the mentioning of connections has been exhausted quickly, one can ask clients if they would like to listen to the noted statements again in a kind of meditation. If this is affirmed, one reads the notes slowly aloud. Sometimes this results in something like a small poetic text that awakens new associations.

If the connections found have been written down on a flipchart sheet, the client can be asked to let his eyes wander again slowly from top to bottom over what has been written. This also elicits comments and additions.

It should be pointed out again at this point that, in this part of the counseling, the participants in the conversation are moving entirely in the realm of the hypothetical. It is about possible connections. We are in a phase of collection, a kind of brainstorming. The mentioned connections might seem very convincing to one person but far-fetched to another. Finally, to a third person, certain answers may even seem absurd and incomprehensible. Any argumentation is therefore out of place. Only with possible concretizations for further proceeding in everyday life ("next step") can arguments and considerations be helpful again. For the time being, it is a matter of fishing for ideas in a sea of possibilities.

Active participation of the counselor

Once several possible connections have been noted, and the client's ideas have been exhausted for the time being, there is the possibility of enriching and detailing individual ones of the mentioned connections with the help of questions. If one wishes to do this, care should be taken to ask open-ended questions as much as possible. "You mentioned XYZ in third place. Can you tell me a little more about that?" Also, at this point, if it seems important, the counselor can bring into the conversation one or two other connections that have occurred to him in the course of the session. We always preface such an intervention with the question "Do you want to hear what has come to mind for me?" Most clients will answer in the affirmative. Such a counselor-added connection should be explicitly presented as a "possible connection." Ideas of the counselor do not take precedence over those of the client in any way.

We are very cautious with this last intervention. It usually seems unnecessary. Implicitly giving the message that "I, the counselor, just see more or more important things than you" should be avoided. However, one author (H.E.) has already experienced the positive effects of such an intervention. For example, out of a whole series of formulated connections, one client spontaneously took up only the one he had mentioned, which proved to be very fruitful.

A next step

Once a list of possible connections has been drawn up and, if necessary, additionally detailed and supplemented, it is a matter of selecting a first and later perhaps also a second item on the list and examining it more closely for its possible meanings:

"PRESERVING THE OPENNESS OF SPACE"

H.W. works in an institution that is mainly preventive but also curative. He has a varied workload, which includes counseling, information work, project management, animation, leading groups, and negotiations with authorities and institutions. In his open, sensitive, but also firm manner, he is well accepted by staff and clients and is very successful in his work overall.

H.W. is particularly burdened by extraordinary tasks at the time of counseling and feels under tremendous time pressure. In addition, he has a paper on his mind that he still has to work on and deliver in a context that is difficult for him. At the same time, he describes a vague, slowly growing disgruntlement and a slight fear of failure that was previously unknown to him.

H.W. formulates as a good result for the counseling session that he can "deal more clearly" with time pressure and learn appropriate strategies. He has a vision for his professional future of a man who can deal with everything that comes his way professionally in a relaxed manner and a good mood. This man has found a good balance in his time management between the demands of his job, those of his family, and his own interests.

In the decentering phase, the counselor asks H.W. to demarcate an "appropriate space" on the floor with adhesive strips without telling him what this space will be used for. Then he is given the task of laying out a mosaic within eight minutes using rectangular pieces of paper of different sizes and colors—from large sheets of drawing paper to small Post-it notes. The room is clearly too large for such a task, which presents a special challenge for the client.

This is a particular form of task setting. H.W. is already quite familiar with decentering. He is an ambitious man who loves challenges. The counselor wanted to leave it up to chance and H.W. to determine the level of challenge. While for many clients it is essential to create a loving, protected, and safe arrangement for decentering, challenging tasks can be very beneficial for specific clients.

After a short hesitation, H.W. sets to work and carefully lays out a small figure in one part of the room. When this is finished, and it becomes obvious that he cannot continue like this in the time available, he begins to lay curved, generously interrupted lines with the smaller Post-it notes under time pressure. In this way, he can cope with the dimensions of the room and also manages to keep to the given time limit to some extent. In the end, the small figure is integrated into freely placed, wide, curved lines, which creates interior spaces, small agglomerations, and generous openings to the outside.

The aesthetic analysis (Section 4.7) brings in a short time a lot of details about the created work and the process that led to its creation.

After a total of about 25 minutes, both sit back in the counseling chairs, and the counselor asks about possible connections between what was created in the decentering phase and what was said about it, and all that was talked about at the beginning of the session. H.W. knows this question, which introduces the harvesting phase, from previous sessions and gets right to it: "The openness; being able to leave a room without being afraid." "You have to take the curve." "As soon as you leave the big sheets, something else comes. That these [pointing to the little Post-it notes] embody something so light, moving, open." "Looking at the whole makes the beginning [meaning the small figure he started with and took a relatively long time to create] seem banal. What was in focus at the beginning is no longer significant."

It is evident that H.W.'s remarks have no direct relation to the wording of the concern as it had been expressed at the beginning of the session. Also, as stated, it is too early at this point for reference to the concern.

Since the time available is usually not sufficient to go into all the mentioned connections in more detail, we usually let one or two be selected in order to deepen them—for the time being, still on the associative level. How the selection of the connections to be worked on is made varies. Often, we let the client choose by asking, for example, "Of these various possible connections that have come to mind, which one interests you the most?" Occasionally, the counselor himself selects one of the connections mentioned: "Is it OK if we look at this point a little more closely?" A combination of the two approaches is also possible: "You are most interested in this possible connection. I would still be interested in the one you mentioned last. Let's look at both of them a little more closely!"

H.W. is free to choose and names the second-mentioned connection ("taking the curve") first and then the first-mentioned ("openness").

We start with the aspect "taking the curve": "If this aspect would turn out to be an important connection between what happened in the studio room and what you said at the beginning of the session, what could it all be?" H.W. relates his thoughts to the desired balance in time management: "...that you can take this [the curve to balance]... there is movement in it...but there are centrifugal forces, that is, new forces are at work. You have to be mindful if you want to take the curve well."

On the "openness" aspect, H.W. mentions that the openings to the outside that can be seen in his lines are exactly in the two places where there are actually doors in the workspace. "The doors are there—and they are open."

The role of the counselor in this part of the counseling is preferably passive. He listens, tries to understand the client's train of thought, perhaps asks questions, and takes notes. Only very rarely can it be helpful to point out a detail in the artistic design in a questioning way. The point is to allow the client to pursue her thoughts undisturbed and to express freely the hypotheses, associations, and speculations that arise. In this phase of the conversation, however, most clients express their thoughts not so much speculatively and hypothetically as in a way that makes it seem likely that they themselves are convinced of their conclusiveness. Once in a while, however, a client expresses self-doubt, saying that she is unsure whether what she is saying is a "real connection." Our almost stereotypical response to such a remark is that no one can know at this point. Only later would it become clear to what extent something mentioned was or was not a "real" and important connection.

Solutions of the second order

What is harvested usually turns out to be a "solution of the second order" in the further course of the work with a client. This metaphorical term is meant to indicate that what is found during the harvest usually does not contain direct instructions for action for the concern formulated at the beginning of the session, which could be called a "first-order solution." What is harvested has a different quality, is more fundamental, more general. Sometimes one even has the impression that clients formulate life wisdom in a more or less coded, metaphorical language. However, they do not seem to be aware of this at all. They are merely trying to find possible connections between what was going on in the decentering and the situation as it had come up in the previous part of the conversation. Since, logically, there cannot be any connections between these two things, they are free to give space to their ideas.

H.W. chose the aspect "taking the curve" for deepening. This is an expression that is popular in Switzerland, especially among young people. It probably comes from motorcycle racing and means something like "to behave skillfully in a difficult but manageable situation." For H.W., who had ridden a motorcycle himself in his youth, the focus may therefore have been on the fact that the balance he wanted to achieve in time management was a difficult undertaking that could not necessarily develop predictable centrifugal forces. In following up, his conclusion is "You have to be mindful if you want to take the curve well." Further, he also talks about sometimes "slowing down" and being aware "that there's a curve coming now."

The ideas about the aspect "openness" seem to indicate that H. W. could pay more attention to the opportunities and possibilities that arise in his situation and from his tasks.

Based on these and further thoughts on the two aspects, "taking the curve" and "openness," the counselor and client discuss some concrete consequences for H.W.'s everyday work. Finally, the counselor asks to what extent the "good result" formulated at the beginning of the session has been achieved. H.W. says: "It has not been achieved directly.

But something else has been achieved: making the whole thing more relaxed. To maintain this openness of space."

If what is put into language in the harvesting conversation phase is something like second-order solutions in the sense mentioned above (i.e., they have a more fundamental, general quality), it follows that it is necessary to relate the corresponding statements to the client's everyday life. Only then can concrete solution steps be formulated.

Integration

In the final stage of integration, the counselor's assistance may be necessary and important. Quite often, however, clients are effortlessly able to formulate concrete steps themselves that can be derived from their statements on harvesting. This is shown by the next example:

"TREADING IN THE VOID"

M. is a young career counselor who started her first job in the profession a few weeks ago. In the foreground of one of the first coaching sessions are advice-seekers who leave M. with the feeling of "treading in the void." As an example, she tells of Claude, a 30-year-old man who, after graduating from high school, dropped out of a first-degree program after four years without graduating, which was then repeated after two years in a different field of study. After a period of working in his parents' business, he started his own company, which went bankrupt after a relatively short time. Currently, Claude is in a postgraduate course of study, which is not very satisfying for him. What proves to be particularly difficult for M. is that the man appears very suave and confident, and presents himself as a "man of the world." M. has the impression of not being able to approach this client, which gives her the aforementioned feeling of "treading in the void." In the coaching session, M. would like to get input on what she should pay attention to with Claude in the upcoming meetings.

The harvest from the decentering phase yields two results that are important to M.: (a) "a new dimension has been added"; (b) a striking contrast between "soft" and "hard." Here M. connects "soft" with respect to Claude with "taking in, listening" and "hard" with "taking clear positions and reflecting them back, even if they are unpleasant."

Due to time constraints, only one of these second-degree solutions can be worked on further in the integration phase. M. chooses point (a).

The coach asks M. what this "new dimension" could mean in concrete terms in the next meeting with Claude. It is immediately clear to her that it means "going deeper." Together, they discuss various possibilities of "going deeper." The coach also contributes his own professional reflections. It is about different forms of diagnostic recording of Claude's situation, about forms of leading the conversation, and about contents of the conversation that had not or had hardly been discussed so far. From the various possibilities, M. selects those points that seem important, urgent, and feasible for her. At the end of the discussion phase, a small plan of action is drawn up, which is to form the basis of the subsequent discussion with Claude.

Client's own activity

One might ask whether, in this example, the decentering and its reappraisal were at all meaningful and necessary. Couldn't the coach have asked specific questions to clarify everything M. has done with Claude so far and then highlight and evaluate what was missing and outline the next steps with her?

We think that this would have been a possible way. However, it must be kept in mind that with such a procedure, the coach very easily gets into the role of teacher and lecturer, which M. has become sufficiently familiar with during her training in recent years. At least implicitly, M. is told that in such an approach the coach is the one who "knows it," who finds out what has gone unnoticed, and then tells the client what to do. The client is thrust into the role of the student. This is not bad in principle but does little for professional independence and security.

Our approach conveys other implicit messages. The decentering action lets M. experience the independent mastering of an unexpected, previously unpracticed task. In the present example (it was a simple installation task), M. spontaneously expressed her astonishment during the aesthetic analysis at the short time in which she had succeeded in achieving an appealing result, "although such tasks are not my thing." From this sense of achievement, she then formulated hypothetical connections to the initial situation and selected one of them that seemed meaningful to her at the moment or otherwise interested her specifically. Finally, with the coach's help, she formulated a plan for how to proceed.

M. herself was active in all parts of the process described. The insights gained came from her, even though she might not have been able to specify in detail how she came to them. She had the experience that—within the given framework and under the guidance of the coach—she was able to tackle the described problem herself. The implicit message of the approach in this session could have been: "Even as a beginner, I am capable of finding viable solutions myself." Perhaps even: "I am capable of more than I have thought so far. I can trust myself to do more."

Accordingly, our approach not only strengthens (professional) self-confidence but also awakens curiosity and the joy of discovery. The mixture between creative and surprising conversation phases and those that are clearly structured is training and a model for many newcomers to the profession as to how they could approach their tasks themselves without necessarily having to adopt the method of Intermodal Decentering. This became very clear in the further course of work with M.

For once, leave the "next step" open

The integration phase is undoubtedly an important part. Now there are not so rare situations where, after the harvest with its sometimes almost sibylline second-degree solutions, detailed integration work with a careful formulation of procedural steps is not indicated. Sometimes we have the impression that it is even a hindrance to successfully dealing with the problem to discussing "next steps" in concrete terms.

"FREEDOM" OR "MORNING DAWN ON THE BALTIC SEA"

E. comes to coaching sessions because of professional issues. On one occasion, she asks to be allowed to make an exception to this. The single mother wants to bring up the issue involving her 21-year-old son, which has been bothering her for a very long time. The son still lives at home. Asked for a possible title for her problem story, she says, "Always the same."

It is the story of the older of two sons, who as a toddler delighted his mother with his imagination and self-confidence, touched her in kindergarten and in the first years of school with his intense theatrical play, but in adolescence became increasingly difficult for the single mother. School difficulties, theft in the home, later drug use, which today coincides with unemployment and a lifestyle that contrasts with the one she cultivated at home—all this causes E. great concern. She reports that she had been enormously committed to this child for years. However, she also became increasingly entangled in her son's problems. An attempt to distance herself, combined with her insistence on a few house rules, had more or less failed. Again and again, she gets involved in lengthy discussions. Time and again, she also agrees to compromises. Afterward, it often turned out that she had been lied to.

As a good result of the consultation, E. expects "to have an idea to try something different."

Decentering consists of an installation on a small table with a limited number of objects. The installation is then intermodally supplemented with a haiku. E. gives the entire work the title "Freedom." The brief aesthetic analysis yields some clear statements, and in the harvesting phase, E. can name a whole list of possible connections to the initial conversation.

E. would like to take a closer look at and deepen the possible relationship between the title she found for her work "Freedom" and her situation. She experiences this reference as a feeling. She cannot describe the feeling with words at the moment, but an image comes to her mind. It is early morning, long before sunrise. She is standing on a seashore. Slowly, the dawn begins to rise over the sea. It is a hazy day, so that the dividing line between sky and water is blurred. The slowly rising light, by no means radiant but perceptibly growing stronger, produces a variety of color effects. From the front, rather than from the right, there is some movement in the sea. It is as if the light and the water were playing with each other...

E. is obviously fascinated by the image. The coach asks her to describe the image in all its detail and then its effect on the viewer. Additional questions, which all refer to the surface of the picture or the scene (differences in the play of colors in the right half of the picture compared to the left, changing movements in the sea, etc.), reveal further details.

The concluding intervention of the session consists only in the coach's remark that the image and its atmosphere could represent something like a gauge of what is important for E. in her current life situation.

From a whole list of possible connections between the decentering event and her everyday situation, E. chose the word "freedom." She was not able to articulate the connection in words. She also did not want to translate the feeling she was ultimately concerned with into everyday language but described, quasi-metaphorically, a scene by the sea. Through his questions, the counselor helped E. to describe this scene in great detail, creating a very intimate atmosphere in the room. The counselor then decided to close the session on this emotional high point. His final intervention with the indirect task was intended to make it easier for E. to recall and, if need be, to use at home the image of what "freedom" meant to her.

Continuing the conversation "according to the rules" by discussing in detail a "next concrete step" would probably have destroyed the magic that had been created in the consultation room by the description of the scene by the sea. Therefore, the session was concluded at this point, and the date for the next one was agreed upon.

In the next session, after a six-week summer break, E. reported a fundamental change in her behavior towards her son, which in turn influenced his behavior. Her connection with him had clearly improved. Her usual reminding behavior had disappeared. Instead, short, good conversations resulted more often. "My ears are not so strained wide open anymore. The relationship with him has become so ordinary. I'm just there." Recently, the son even suggested going out to dinner together. This meal then also took place "and I listened to him with growing interest."

In response to the counselor's related question, E. remarks that the image of the beginning of the day by the sea had accompanied her throughout. "The image kept coming to my mind. It was like a touchstone for what I was looking for." She could use it to measure how close she was to what was important to her in her behavior towards her son. (All that was important had been summed up in the phrase "freedom" in the last session.)

Inquiry two months later revealed that the connection with the

> son had temporarily deteriorated again, but she was now able to keep herself out of it much better.

The example makes it clear. We do propose a specific procedure for the discussion phase of the harvest. This also proves successful. However, in our process-oriented approach, the process that is happening with the client takes precedence. If it becomes clear that something important is going on with her, it makes sense to be guided by this. And this is true even if, as in the example of M., the professional has only a very vague idea of what the desired new behavior might be about.

In general, the more familiar someone is with the standard sequence of the conversation, the more freely they can deal with its individual parts.

Open questions and a curious, waiting attitude

Shaping the harvesting phase is not easy for beginners: What is required is an appreciative, curious, and open mindset. This includes waiting and leaving the verbalization of the content entirely up to the client. However, it also means taking the lead in the conversation in a friendly, determined manner if, for example, the client wants to go on a rambling justification of a connection she has found or wants to abort the search for other associations too hastily.

This required mindset is also manifested in question forms that are as open as possible and which follow the client's choice of words.

> P. chooses for the detail processing "tackling the aggression" that has become visible for him in the decentering. Open questions about this could be: "Can you tell me something more about this?" "Specifically, what did you find to be 'aggressive'?" "And how do you see the connection to your everyday situation?" "Does this apply to both the aggressive and the tackling?"
>
> In contrast, we often encounter questions from beginners in the training situation such as "Did you feel aggressive throughout?" "When did you feel more aggressive—at the beginning or at the end?" "Do you experience such destructive sides [P. tore something during his paper sculpture, but never used the word 'destroy' or 'destructive' himself]) in yourself on other occasions?" Closed questions phrased

> in this way direct attention in a particular direction and exclude other possibilities. Often they could be answered with a simple yes or no. By their very wording, they detract from the richness of the harvest.
>
> Of course, a question is not made more open by the fact that the counselor herself provides various possible answers: "Did you feel yourself to be very aggressive or only moderately aggressive?"
>
> An open question forces the client to think for himself and encourages him to search and discover for himself. This fosters a conversational climate of curiosity and openness to the surprising. And this is exactly what is required in this phase of the conversation.

In the same direction as the closed or too strongly focused questions, there is a tendency to limit the initial question for the harvest. For example, what happened and what emerged in the decentering phase is compared with the initially formulated concern, and this concern is possibly repeated word for word. Or only the "final product" of the decentering is focused on—for example, the last take of a musical improvisation—and the whole process that led to it and the "intermediate products" are disregarded.

We think that in order to find lasting solutions, it is important to compare the whole situation in the meeting chairs—that is, everything that went on at the beginning of the session—with everything that happened and emerged during the decentering.

It also seems important to us to maintain the client's choice of words during the phase of collecting and concretizing hypothetical associations. Often, on the other hand, the following happens. Supervisee: "I'll bring that up right away next time and I will not wait until..." Supervisor: "You mean that you now have the courage to be concrete the next time...?" This type of slight rephrasing by the professional may be helpful or even important later in the integration phase. However, during the gathering, concretizing, and deepening of possible relationships, we try to avoid it. Here, the weightings and nuances should be entirely determined by the client. In concrete terms, this means that we largely adopt the client's wording for our questions and comments.

In summary, it can be said that the discussion phase of the harvest places high demands on the counselor. During this phase, she must structure and direct clearly, at the same time leaving the client to take the lead in terms of content. This goes so far that any rephrasing should be avoided in this stage of the conversation.

What can be harvested appears in the form of associations, vague conjectures, hypotheses, and ideas that are difficult to understand, occasionally, but in formulations of relatively plausible connections. We speak of "second-order solutions," and by this we mean that, in these statements, we can find hints to what is behind, to what has been overlooked so far, to what is fundamental. It is therefore important to first collect a larger number of such assumptions. One or two of these assumptions should then be selected for the recording of the possible meanings and the integration into everyday reality. It may be surprising that clients often choose the most incomprehensible, abstruse idea for further processing.

The conversation during the harvest, at least in the gathering phase, moves in the airy, "bottomless" height of free associations. This is unusual and requires the participants to be tolerant of what emerges.

Harvesting takes time. One cannot start after a long phase of decentering in the last five minutes of the available time. If you ever find yourself under such time pressure, you are advised to combine harvesting with a "homework" assignment or postpone it until the next session.

The associations from harvesting will hardly ever directly answer the questions included in the formulated concern. Further processing is required. This happens in the conversation section called "integration," where conclusions for everyday life can be drawn. Mostly, however, it is helpful to contribute something additional as a counselor, which can support the sustainable continuation of what has been elaborated upon.

4.9 Sustainable continuation

A single session usually lasts no more than one and a half hours. If it is counseling or therapy, it may be 3–7 days before the next session. If it is supervision or coaching, it may be longer. In any case, the time outside the therapy or counseling session is many times longer than the session time itself. In this case, it is often appropriate to give the participants something to take home with them from the session, in the sense of a continuation of the work that has been started.

Instructions, assignments, suggestions

This something can be concrete. Clients who have painted, drawn, or written in the decentering phase always wish to take their work or document home. An installation can be photographed and then taken home. As was shown in Chapter 3, the artistic work, as it is experienced and in its substantial presence, has the quality of something existential. This is true not only in the phase of extraordinary reality within the session; it can retain this quality in the client's everyday life as well. This makes it possible to consider works or parts of a work created during a decentering phase as helping spirits that can have an effect on the client's life.

> Z. is asked to take the small figure that has become particularly meaningful to her during an installation work home and place it there in an "appropriate place" until the next session.
>
> In a similar vein, the counselor encourages M. to carry a small stone from the stone sculpture created during decentering with her until the next session. It is small enough to fit easily in a trouser pocket or a small handbag.

The creative activity can be assigned like dream and daydream to a metabolic area of the soul and metaphorically called soul nourishment. Like the nutritional substance in the physical realm, soul nourishment can be used as a kind of medicine or as a means of psychic dietetic. Dietetics (Greek: *diaita*) regulate the way of living healthily.

In the counseling process, these considerations could be concretized—for example, as follows: "Sing one or more times a day when you are alone at work instead of turning on the radio!" Or: "Maybe place this self-made instrument in such a place that your gaze falls on it when you doubt yourself again!" Here is a concrete example:

> A. (who will be discussed later) encountered the phenomenon of lightness in the harvest phase of a decentering process. When asked about sources of lightness in her everyday life, A. mentions her partner.

The counselor encourages her to place an object that reminds her of him in the counseling room. Together, they then ponder the most favorable places to position this object.

Such instructions can be given in a direct or indirect form, depending on the situation. Or it makes sense to design them as an assignment or homework.

"EMBEDDING THE UNDESIRABLE"

C. is in the process of setting up a consulting practice after working as an employee for many years. She reports that she allows herself to be put under time pressure by clients and has a tendency to justify and legitimize her own interventions or suggestions that may be not quite commonplace during the session or—conversely—to quickly withdraw them if there are signs of hesitation or reluctance on the part of the client. She is very annoyed by this behavior, which she perceives as a devaluation of her consulting style that is developing. In the future, she wishes to be able to feel a "ground of serenity and confidence within herself and to remain in this basic feeling during a counseling session."

In the harvesting phase after decentering, C. is most surprised by a rather weighty stone. When selecting objects for the installation proposed by the counselor, she had associated this stone with the feeling that led to each case of the undesirable behavior in her practice. Now, at the conclusion of the design work, it merely appears at the edge of the installation, embedded in soft fabric. Asked about a possible reference to everyday work, she says, "I could sense this feeling as embedded...it's not so alone anymore...I should take care of all my feelings...almost tenderly." And concluding, "I would like to pursue this view a little more, that it might be able to expand in a way."

It is natural for the counselor in such a situation to echo the client's spontaneously expressed intention. He did so in this case in the following way: "I suggest that you follow up on this experience and the thoughts associated with it a bit in the context of half an hour before the next time. In doing so, also think about what supports the 'embedding' of the unwanted feelings in you. And [with a wink] if you also want to concretize this supportive aspect artistically in the sense of an experiment [C. works with her clients partly in an art-oriented way], then this is, of course, also OK."

Ten days later, C. brings two self-painted pictures into the session, which can be profitably worked with further.

The good effect of a homework assignment is supported if the counselor, as in C.'s case, takes up expressions or metaphors that the client has expressed spontaneously in the session itself in the instruction for the assignment.

In C's example, part of the assignment was formulated in terms of a task. If it is about deepening or enriching goals, newly discovered behaviors, or feelings, the term "experiment" is preferable to "task." This makes the situation more open and gives clients opportunities for initiative and new discoveries. Tasks, especially those labeled "homework," often have a bad connotation for clients. The memories of school days and homework are too strong. For this reason alone, "homework" should be given sparingly.

An experiment to explore what is desirable

We have very good experiences when something new or desirable, discovered for the first time in the session, can be enriched by a new medium at home in the sense of an experiment.

"THE SQUARE AND THE SOFT"

A. is a newcomer to the profession. In the second supervision session, the conversation turns to two very different approaches taken by the young counselor. One is very determined and wants to achieve a concrete result quickly. A. knows this behavior very well from her previous job. The second, which is beginning to emerge, is more hesitant, apparently more process-oriented. A. is bad at describing this second side, so the counselor suggests exploring the two sides in a drawing/painting way. A. emphasizes that she "can't draw at all" but then tries. For the familiar behavior, an angular structure is created, which A. calls "The Double Arrow." For the still little-known behavior, a round, quite sweeping, upwardly open structure is created with the title "The Electric Cables." A. is surprised that, contrary to her intention, picture 1 extends much less far up to the upper edge of the picture than picture

2. Her associations with picture 1 are: "angular, straight, clear, narrow." For image 2, they are: "round, soft, free, open."

To further explore the two sides and explore their meaning and scope, the counselor suggests an experiment. A. should bring to the next session a piece of music or part of a piece of music for each of these two sides that she likes and appeals to her.

The next time, A. does not bring any recordings with her but says she has the music clearly in her head. She can then describe the two pieces of music in detail to the counselor. For picture 1, it is the march of a brass band; for picture 2, melodiously flowing meditation music. The aesthetic analysis of this fantasized music succeeds only rudimentarily. On the other hand, A. can connect the two pieces with some experiences that are important for her. The theme of the two different styles of counseling, which ultimately also embody different lifestyles for A., is present throughout the entire supervision work with this client over a year and a half.

Enrichment

Solution- and resource-oriented work repeatedly encounters the fact that counselors and clients can usually talk about problems and conflicts in much greater detail and nuance than about strengths and abilities. The familiar questions of the classical solution-oriented approach increase attention to the conditions of success. De Shazer and Berg (cited in de Jong and Berg, 1998) have additionally emphasized the importance of detailed descriptions of a good future. They speak of "goals" and "noticing what clients want." Our approach tries with some success to capture these sides of our clients' lives through specific questions.

The inclusion of artistic forms of expression opens up further possibilities here, broadening and deepening them from the point of view of psychological experience. We speak of "enrichment" in this context. To enrich a positive vision of the future or a successful exceptional behavior means to make it more richly experienced in its various nuances and from different perspectives. This is quite possible by asking appropriate questions within everyday language. Artistic media, however, reveal exceptional potential in this field.

As in the example of A., those who can (also) express the desired new style of counseling musically or in the form of a non-representational picture they have painted themselves thus also grasp sides of the soul that possibly elude everyday language. In addition, there is the already mentioned nurturing aspect of artistic expression. Here we start from the assumption that a self-created work with aesthetic appeal is more effective—that is, more "nourishing"—than the consumptive handling of the artistic work of others.

Subjecting artistic works taken with them to an aesthetic analysis

If the counselor suggests such experiments and tasks or carries them out in the session itself, the procedures and principles already described in Intermodal Decentering (Sections 4.6 and 4.7) apply. It is about the art or the work, and not at all about an illustrative or symbolic representation of experiences. The more it is possible to devote oneself completely to the creative process, the more the counselor's instruction facilitates this devotion and the richer will be the harvest afterward. We have become accustomed, analogous to the procedure of Intermodal Decentering, to carry out an aesthetic analysis of every work that is brought from home, be it self-made or selected—that is, to work out a careful description "on the surface." On the part of the counselor, this requires a specific repertoire of adequate questions, on the part of the client often some training in generating a particular vocabulary, and on the part of both a good amount of patience.

Following such an aesthetic analysis of homework, it is useful to capture the momentary meaning of what has been formed or experienced in everyday language and, if necessary, to make a connection between it and certain aspects of the question or of one's own life. An artistic creation alone or immersion in another's artwork may have nourishing effects in the sense of soul sustenance; as a rule, however, its effect in promoting and supporting concrete steps towards a solution is likely to be insufficient. Together, however, the artistic experience and its verbalization have the desired positive effects.

Attentive readers guess correctly: trying out such continuations of the work started in the counseling and therapy room was strongly encouraged by de Shazer and Berg (de Jong and Berg, 1998). Similar to these two pioneers of the solution-focused approach to work (Berg, oral communication, 2003), we most often employ forms of observational tasks. In the rare cases where we propose a behavioral task, we set it in a completely open form and like to combine it with playful guidance. An example of such guidance in a combination of observation and behavioral task might be:

> Until we meet again in two weeks, flip a coin each night for the next five nights. If "heads" appears, then spend the following working day as you always do. However, if "tails" appears, then do something different the following day. Next time, report back to me how you did. And if you have the misfortune that only "heads" appears, then I'll allow you to flip the coin again or even two at a time until "tails" shows up.

In contrast to de Shazer and Berg, we very often incorporate design elements into the tasks and experiments. Some of the examples already described illustrate this. Likewise, we by no means give a task after each session, as the classical solution-oriented approach to work suggests. In certain situations, it even seems counterproductive to us to end the session with a task. The decentering process of E., described in Section 4.8, shows such a situation. The magic and intensity of the imagination on the topic of freedom would probably have been destroyed or at least impaired by both a discussion of concrete steps and a homework assignment.

It seemed more important to the counselor to let E. leave the session in her emotional state at that time so that it could continue to have an effect for as long as possible. That this approach was appropriate was shown by the subsequent conversation after the summer break, during which E. mentioned that the imagined picture had been with her throughout and, we can conclude, effectively supported the positive behavioral changes.

Uncompleted assignments

What seems fundamentally important to us is the way of dealing with unfinished tasks, to which de Shazer (oral communication, *c.*1999) already drew attention. A task that is not done or a task that has been misunderstood or is done in a different way for other reasons is by no means a sign of "noncompliance" or even resistance. It is nothing more or less than feedback to the counselor. The task did not fit. Maybe the task was given too early; maybe the client could not or would not go for it for some other reason. It is not essential to understand the meaning of this feedback in detail. But it is important to take it seriously as the work progresses.

From time to time, a task not completed can still be put to use beneficially.

THE "CIRCLING" BREAKS OUT

V., a coach and team consultant who is quite successful as a freelancer, has for years been repeatedly afflicted by periods of feeling down and doubtful. V. calls this state "circling." The circling not only occupies him mentally; it also affects him physically, makes him tight, takes his breath away, and emotionally takes all his courage. In the discussions, it becomes clear that V. is faced with many exceptional situations and has developed in part successful strategies for overcoming these. In the fourth session, rudiments of a not exclusively negative description of "circling" appear for the first time. The counselor, therefore, suggests that V., who is occasionally active musically and as a watercolor painter in his free time, could give "circling" an artistic form at home and bring it with him in a suitable form to the next session.

In the next session, V. says that the task "fell out of his mind" but that he could actually paint the circles, and spontaneously remarks: "I see the picture right in front of me." This sentence leads the counselor to work with the non-existent picture in the manner of virtual decentering—that is, to treat "the picture" as if it were lying there, and thus to carry out an aesthetic analysis and a phase of harvesting.

This approach works exceptionally well. V. finds previously unimagined resources in the virtual picture and subsequently also several possible references to his everyday work. He intends to paint "the picture, or a reproduction of it" by the next session.

This next session takes place only after a longer interruption since V. has taken a previously planned sabbatical of several weeks in the meantime. V. brings photographs of two self-painted watercolors to this session. One shows the discussed picture, and the second one represents how the circling has changed in the meantime. V. reports

> that the last session became very important for him. While painting, the main insight for him was "Hey, circling is colorful!" And about the second painting, he says: "Here the colorfulness has broken out, and it can't be tamed anymore." At this same session, V. reports so many positive changes that counselor and client jointly conclude to end the coaching work at this point. The conclusion is unexpected for both but feels coherent.

Of course, such a course is not typical for our approach. However, it clearly shows that even a task that has not been done can have an extremely positive effect. One condition for this is presumably that the forgotten or differently completed task is not treated like an incorrectly completed school task, but that it is taken seriously as feedback and that one is able to continue in a process-oriented manner.

As a rule, we always construct follow-on tasks and experiments anew, regardless of what was once suggested in earlier sessions. However, it may be useful for certain questions to tie a subsequent task to an earlier one. One reason for this would be to savor a sense of achievement one more time.

Somewhat different was the situation of C. described earlier in this section. Her problem proved to be a fundamental attitude toward herself and others. Her great willingness to work on the topic made it useful to coordinate the homework over several sessions. Thus, parallel to working on current issues, working on the fundamental issue raised in a kind of exploration and training program was possible.

In summary, experiments and continuing tasks carried out at home not only have a bridging function between the counseling and therapy sessions but can continue the process started in the practice room in the everyday context of the client. In addition, they allow the progress of the work done together to be illustrated visually in an easily verifiable way.

5

Fundamental Reflections on Language, Art, and Play

This chapter summarizes some fundamental aspects of the use of language and the approach to art and play that are typical of our practice and are important to us. In doing so, we do not limit ourselves to enumerating and presenting these aspects but put them in context with the theoretical, philosophical, and artistic foundations that guide our actions.

5.1 On the use of language

Counselors encounter the reality of their clients primarily through language. In the verbal message, people seeking help try to make the facts of their world understandable to the other person. We all know that this can only succeed to some extent. Even more important is the fact that something that is put into language and communicated to someone else becomes a social construction. This construction involves the actors who are present, but possibly also those who are not present—the client as speaker, the counselor as listener and questioner, other important reference persons—and, last but not least, cultural backgrounds, which are important within the situation that is brought up for discussion. In a given conversational situation, this is easily overlooked. If the other person is credible, we usually take what is reported to us at face value.

The counselor must remember that she always influences the reality with which she is dealing in counseling. This reality, as it appears in counseling, is the product of a process of negotiation—primarily guided by language. In other words, the story that is told and emerges anew in the course of the conversation is co-determined in tone and its general orientation by the concretely and virtually present (see also Bürgi and Eberhart, 2004, chapter 6).

At first glance, this may seem annoying, irritating, and disruptive. However, if you take a closer look at it, it turns out to be an opportunity.

The language in the counseling or therapy room can construct reality anew

In counseling and therapy scenarios—and, of course, in other conversational situations as well—reality appears as a socially constructed reality mediated by language. It is not the event itself that is reported that is central, but the meaning that is attributed to this event. This circumstance opens up great possibilities for the counseling and therapeutic conversation. By speaking to each other in a particular way in the protected setting of the consulting room, there is the possibility of finding new, additional meanings that allow reality to appear in a new light. To put it more precisely and pointedly: the otherness of the language used in the counseling and therapy room constructs reality anew.

In contrast to the logical-argumentative language (Bruner, 1986) cultivated in the sciences, in conversation, meanings are mostly embedded in stories. Here, it is not primarily precisely defined terms, stringent logic, and freedom from contradiction that are required, but plausibilities—such as emotional logic, emotional concern, and coherence of meaning. If these qualities are present, the story is convincing.

This means that every story can be understood as a system. The individual parts are in connection with each other and influence each other. The story as a whole makes sense, which can present itself as truth. Stories organize the experiences of the teller and give them meaning (e.g., Anderson and Goolishian, 1990). When a story is told, it is also influenced by the listeners—in other words, by the context.

Humans live in stories. Narrative language is, so to speak, the natural language of human beings. These stories provide us with the structure with which we can appropriately reduce the complexity of the world and thus make it livable and communicable.

People identify with their stories

Clients' stories are often problem-saturated—that is, what is reported is repeatedly brought into connection with the problem at the center. In this sense, they are repetitive and comparatively poor in content. Surprises are rarely found. As a rule, experiences that do not correspond to the view of the problem are not taken into account and are not included in the story told.

However, humans are fundamentally "multi-storied"—that is, they are usually able to narrate a given event from different perspectives. In contrast to this usual behavior towards one's own stories, problem stories have a tendency to freeze.

This circumstance has a disastrous effect because the stories a person tells about himself have an effect back on him.

Humans identify with their stories, especially those that they tell over and over again. Thus, one can say that an illness story that is told over and over again ultimately fixes the person in question in her being ill. An illness that one talks about with oneself and with others becomes a social phenomenon. One then no longer reacts only to the scientific fact of illness but above all to the social phenomenon. This can be disastrous, for example, in the case of chronic illnesses, since verbalization usually acts as objectification (von Schlippe and Lob-Corzilius, 1993; Stierlin, 1990). The latter, however, can also have a positive effect on the sufferer's state of mind—if, for example, analogous to Alcoholics Anonymous, they repeatedly confess their situation publicly and support each other in self-help groups. This acts as a kind of reconciliation with the condition that has been declared irreversible and can be very relieving under certain circumstances.

In the opposite way, this process can also be observed in solution and success stories. These emphasize healthy and successful experiences. Clients begin to pay more attention to these sides and eventually make them parts of their own self-image.

Stories that a person tells about himself, therefore, have real effects on his life. They change his reality. From such a point of view, human life can be understood as a process of telling and retelling stories. The meanings that one's actions acquire for a person, and the ideas, thoughts, and images that he has of himself, are bound up in his narratives. However, physical conditions, culture, social structure, and the concrete effects of one's actions also set limits on the effects of the stories that are told.

It has been argued that meanings are socially and interpersonally constructed. In the interpersonal sphere, meanings arise when two or more people understand the same occurrence in the same way. They then begin to speak, as we say in everyday life, "the same language" and confirm each other's meaning. Seen in this way, meaning is identical with (the same) understanding. This understanding is context-bound and never valid across all times. According to Anderson and Goolishian, "understanding is always 'on the way,' provisional, and never fully attainable" (1990, p.222). In this process, interlocutors ultimately understand only the descriptions and explanations, not the events themselves.

Newly found meanings are fragile. They must be acquired again and again in conversation. If they are to become and remain behaviorally effective, they must also be tacitly or explicitly accepted by the relevant people in the environment. Michael White (1997) speaks of the fact that newly found meanings—he calls them "alternative stories"—must not only be linked to clients' previous lives, intentions, and goals but should also be told onwards.

Sometimes the latter is only possible to a very limited extent because the current significant others are not interested in what is about to happen. They have become familiar with the client's previous (suffering) state, and have arranged themselves accordingly. Systemically speaking, an over-stable equilibrium has been established in the social environment, which is difficult to unhinge. In this situation, there is often nothing for the client to do but to "emigrate" from his previous environment. People have to learn to determine who should belong to their (life) circle and who they have to withdraw membership from.

The presentation of our methodological approach in Chapter 4 shows that we take these considerations into account in many parts without adopting the procedure of White's "narrative systems approach" in detail. Already in the clarification of the assignment, but especially in the articulation of goal visions and a good outcome for the current session, we carefully record what the client is striving for, what is important to him, and what he longs for. During the problem recording, the problem-free times are also important to us. Here, the first approaches to alternative narratives already show up.

The resource-oriented questioning technique and conversation further contribute to making visible sides of life that put the problem-saturated narrative into perspective. As a rule, the sensorial experience of the artistic work in the decentering phase also makes a central contribution. This sensorial experience of artistic activity, as well as the beauty or a surprising aspect of a work that has been created, touches the client directly and can bring aspects of her own being and corresponding longings into the present that seemed to have disappeared long ago. Finally, the accompaniment of newly discovered and rediscovered feelings and behaviors in everyday life promotes what White understands as "re-telling."

In summary, it can be said that the way language is shaped—that is, the type of dialogue—is of central importance within therapy and counseling. The case studies discussed in the previous chapters, especially in Chapter 4, have made visible in manifold ways how we deal with language. The following thesis-like statements outline the principles and guidelines that guide us.

In therapy, counseling, supervision, and coaching, new stories are looked for that, unlike problem stories, do not diminish and constrict the client's possibilities for action and freedom but rather expand and enrich them. The dialogue or discourse that leads to such narratives is intended to open the connection to what Anderson and Goolishian (1990, p.226) call "the infinite resources of the not-yet-said." In this co-creative process, the counselor is always also co-author of the new story.

Counselors are conversation artists. They are experts in creating a space in which to speak without inhibition and to express something on a probing and trial basis. They are promoters of a discourse in which wonder is articulated through questions, and the answerer does not always and everywhere have to provide proof of the truth of their statements. Counselors speak and ask questions from a position of not knowing. That is, they strive to ensure that their prior experiences and prior knowledge do not blind them to the full meaning of the descriptions of clients' experiences. The position of not knowing is made possible by an attitude of appreciative curiosity. This attitude can be concretized, among other things, by frequent paraphrasing, repeating what is heard in one's own words.

We recommend that our students "watch the client's mouth." Staying in the client's language promotes understanding. An unusual, client-specific expression, for example, can be successfully reused as a metaphor or cipher in later conversational sequences without having to know and understand its meaning in every detail.

Conversely, clients' statements need to be deliberately rephrased—for example, when negative, sometimes even self-punishing expressions are used for positive achievements. In such situations, we believe it is a matter of actual language training, which can effectively support newly discovered or rediscovered attitudes or behaviors.

Similarly, we ask clients to rephrase descriptions of desired behaviors or traits if they have been consistently presented negatively. For example, a 50-year-old client: "I don't want to be so polite and over-correct anymore." "Then how would you like to be?" "I want to be interested. I want to be aware that I am giving him 'my being.'"

We are concerned with promoting a rich everyday language, especially in the areas of skills, strengths, and resources. Often, the focus of clients' attention is on the problem. Successes are taken for granted and are therefore uninteresting. Our questions should help to describe especially these aspects of everyday life in detail: the supporting circumstances, the motives involved, the concrete course of behavior, the accompanying feelings, the kind of satisfaction, the reactions of significant others, etc. The required detailed description sharpens the perception of what is successful and encourages further observations in this field. As a result, gradually, often unnoticed for a longer period of time, one's own narrative and the image that the person in question has of herself also change.

Descriptions should be concrete and specific instead of generalizing. The very concrete and specific description—of a successful action, for example—has an entirely different effect psychologically from a generalizing remark about the same action. Sometimes it is technical jargon, and sometimes it is commonplace phrases ("I just had a good day") or killer phrases ("Yes, yes, I just put my stupid charm to work again") with which clients want to get over something. Friendly, patient, and, at the same time, persistent inquiries help them to remember things more precisely. In the process, aspects can be discovered that were previously—sometimes systematically—overlooked but which often prove very useful as the conversation progresses. This concrete description "on the surface" has nothing to do with an investigative process in which all details have to be brought up in order to get on the trail of the "solution" at best through a seemingly insignificant detail. It has even less to do with jurisprudence, in which facts are gathered to be able to determine "how it really was." Sometimes this is misunderstood by participants in training and professional development.

The importance of a concrete description, which is repeatedly emphasized in this book, is intended to make the richness and the diversity of perspectives of situations—especially of successfully experienced ones—visible. Such a description always proves to be a treasure trove of solutions, and, at the same time, it trains clients to perceive experiences more openly and in a more diverse way.

Descriptions should be concrete instead of abstract. Academics, managers, young doctors, and psychologists sometimes get into the habit of using an abstract repertoire of expressions, which they also apply to themselves in a counseling situation. The abstract formulation helps them to keep a matter at a distance. This can be useful or even necessary in everyday professional life; it is counterproductive in counseling and therapy scenarios. However, for some professionals, it is very difficult and tedious to talk about themselves and their own experiences in a concrete and straightforward way. Here, the artistic or playful activity in the decentering phase and the almost ritually strict, phenomenological, and descriptive mode of expression in the aesthetic analysis can be recreation and training ground at the same time.

Imagination comes up again and again in our conversations. Among other things, it is about the detailed description of desired futures. That is why the subjunctive, as opposed to the indicative, plays an important role. For example, "I want to be able to 'make a point' and not always be rolling around these negative thoughts, like whether the wine I'm going to offer is good enough." "So what would be different if you 'made a point'?" "I would think about what a good life I actually have." "What difference would that make to you?" or "What might an outside person observe about you that would be new to them?"

Likewise, metaphors, images, and possibly poetic forms are usually used more frequently in a conversation that is open to the imagination. People vary in their openness to these forms. Based on the principle that in a counseling situation, the fit of an intervention has to be developed, the counseling process decides whether and to what extent these forms of language come into play or not.

Speech is also used in the artistic or playful phase of decentering. When instructing the decentering activity, the professional uses the logic of everyday language. In the choice of words and formulations, they move within the sensory vocabulary of the corresponding art form. Insofar as speech is also used during artistic activity, the conversation adheres to the language of the respective artistic discipline. This also applies in principle to the aesthetic analysis, which strives for a pure description of what is sensorially perceptible or of what is experienced.

5.2 Art and play

As will be elaborated in Chapter 8, artistic expression is, anthropologically, like language, an existential. The essential differences concern the physical-sensual aspect of art, the strong imaginative component, and the logic of a different kind. One could characterize this logic of a different kind by the fact that it is determined by the senses and is "full of sense" because the logic happens in action (logic of action) and less from a reflection before acting. In artistic activity, one discovers the connections out of the design, so to speak, aesthetically, and less *before* the design, out of an idea.

In the discussions so far, the focus has been on artistic expression. Only occasionally has reference been made to the possibility of play as a form of decentering. In our book, on the other hand, it has been repeatedly mentioned that play procedures can enable decentering in the same way as artistic activity.

If we look at the practice of decentering so far, artistic expression is indeed in the center, and only rarely are play activities applied. It may be true that, in certain situations, it is easier for some people to enter into more or less free play than into artistic activity, which might still be too burdened by the image of the "high and noble" of the arts, respectively by the "right" and "wrong" of art lessons in school. Nevertheless, we must not be deceived here, because often play is too close to the "childish" for clients, and it is then more accessible to enter via folk art, which has replaced the "high and noble" in wider social groups, and this not only in relation to music. To better understand the possibilities of free play in its differences from and overlaps with artistic activity, and also to encourage experimentation with it, we will look at these connections a little more thoroughly below. In doing so, it is helpful to examine the two keywords "play" and "imagination" more closely.

Play

In our language, we are used to using the word "play" when we talk about the arts. For example, "I play music or a musical instrument," "I delight in the play of movement or color of a mobile," or "I attend a play." The root of the word "play" can be found in the ancient Slavic *plesati* or the Gothic *plinsjan*. Both mean "to dance." To play in German—*spielen*—relates to the root *spil*, which we also find in Danish *spille* and Swedish *spel*. Again, the etymological root means "to dance," "to step forward, backward, and sideways," and "to dance in a circle" (Kluge, 1975, p.725). The notion of play is closely connected with dance and the image of the circle. This kinship helps to distinguish play (play) from ruled play (game). The latter is related to "chase" in English.

The term "chase" suggests a directed, linear, goal-oriented "path" towards the prey. The difference between the goal-oriented action of hunting and the circular dance of play can be seen in the different structuring of time. This is linear in directed activities such as hunting but circular in play (Lorenz, 1987, p.395).

In the context of solution-seeking, the principle of enrichment or multi-perspective view and circular questioning is more in line with the notion of circular play space use; linear, on the other hand, is more in line with being linearly focused on the problem to be solved.

For people who play, the satisfaction is in the play itself. This contrasts with the outcome, which is the goal of a rule-based game. In addition, there are many mixed forms; an important form in our work is the play to develop a rules game.

In the context of play range expansion, we have proposed categories of play that can be reduced to the following three (Knill, 1982):

- free play
- rule-based play
- artistic activity or play.

Before we examine these in more detail in relation to practice, let us briefly consider the concept of imagination, for there is neither art nor play in which doing-as-if would not play a role in some way.

Imagination

If we examine the roots of the word "imagination," we find in Latin *imaginatio* and its root *imago*. *Imago*, which could be translated as image, has an extended meaning. According to Meier (1988, p.210), the original linguistic meaning is "in water" or "the thing reflected in water." The word for imagination, *inbilla* in Swedish and *inbilden* in ancient high German, meant something like projecting into the soul.

In our visually oriented society, we are used to reducing imagination to visual images. Because we understand the term *imago* pictorially, we often neglect the other sensory aspects of imagination. In fact, it is not the case that people imagine only in images, but also in sounds, rhythms, movements, courses of action (scenes), spoken messages (dialogues), and inner moving images ("an inner film was playing"), even in smells and tastes ("and there I smelled again the scent of the house where I was on vacation").

This intermodal aspect of imagination, involving different modes of communication, can become important in the enrichment in the course of a session, whether it is about the formulation of a goal or the aesthetic analysis, or an aspect in the phase of harvesting. We then ask not only for imagery. Prompts for other imaginative modalities are also used—for example, "When you describe it to me like this, is there a sound to it?" "Does it also have a smell?" "What kind of music comes to mind?" In aesthetic analysis, where the counselor depends on the memory of a movement or a sequence of sounds to discuss the process, it helps if you can build bridges from another modality: "When you abruptly changed the direction of your dance forward, could you still hear the kind of music that came forth? How was it with the rhythm? With your step?"

Different forms of play and decentering

Every "doing-as-if it were so or otherwise" has a spatial and temporal dimension, the action of each of which can become a play.

We find **free play**, especially with children, in playing with objects to the point of playing something of a scenic nature without prior rules or without a given framework. Free play can also be used in decentering when it is applied as a starting point for a game with rules.

Rule-based play and artistic activity have in common that they determine the play space by rules of a spatial–temporal and material nature. This gives the play a direction towards a result, which in turn leads to a rather linear quality of time.

Artistic activity can be understood as a disciplined play with the imagination, which in its traditional limitations of frame and material (MORE) strives towards a "conclusive work." The work (result) is open and can surprise in its imaginative character. At the same time, this "play" offers a wide range of challenges, the mastering of which must be constantly reinvented.

The **traditional game** is play entirely controlled by rules, the goal of which is known in advance. The outcome is open only insofar as we can achieve the goal more or less efficiently by varying skills. The playing thus offers a challenge known to all, the accomplishment of which depends on skillful strategy and gamesmanship. There is no aesthetic analysis here, only an analysis of strategy and skill. This type of play is well suited to certain educational assignments, but we do not see it in the context of decentering.

The **process of inventing a game** is a way to use the richness of free play in a way that it can be used in decentering. The assignment then also begins with a framework (time, space) and limited material. The order is to play freely with the material until an exciting rule of play emerges that is so satisfying that time is forgotten (circular time). The play (meaning here the result) is open, as, in artistic activity, the work is. This play offers a challenge to be solved innovatively and allows for a kind of aesthetic analysis. The analysis can be done from different perspectives, and the play process offers similar possibilities for reflection as the artistic work process, as we will show in the next section.

5.3 Artistic and playful activity in decentering

We repeatedly hear from clients that they greatly appreciate having a phase without a lot of discussion and language. It is relaxing to focus on things through play, and when they do come up, there is something new that can be addressed together without worrying.

In practice, it has turned out that artistic activity is used in the majority of decentering. This is also true for group work. We suspect that the artistic activity in its essence somehow has the work as a result in mind, even if the process is equally important.

Free play, on the other hand, is already by its nature turned towards the process itself and is not very goal- or work-oriented. It is suitable above all for individual work. Aesthetic analysis, in this case, must focus on the process since the work character is actually expressed in the achievement of a satisfying ludic state. Questions are asked about the actions taken and the arrangements made in the course of the play, and the associated challenges of the person or persons playing the game, as well as everything that was done to achieve that timelessness and fascination that we know from the play: "What interested you most about the play?" "What made you want to change the course of the game?" "When you wanted to give up, what brought you back in?" "What rules you set would you keep next time?"

One could say that in the phase of decentering, free play becomes a kind of performance on objects, in which rules are constantly tried out until it "works" or "works out." In groups, decentering in this way is difficult because rules have to be constantly negotiated in discussions. In such discussions, the problematic easily comes to the fore. We are then in the midst of the problematics of everyday life because of discussions about advantages, sanctions, power, and winning.

When using artistic activity, the question is often raised whether the short time of decentering is sufficient for a reasonable definition of art. We have dealt with this question in the section "Low-skill–high-sensitivity" (see Section 4.6). Here, it is still necessary to point out an effect that is related to the remarks on play.

We observe time and again that full decentering engagement is achieved after only a few minutes if the artistic assignment has a playful character and is limited to simple means, such as shoes in the shoe installation described earlier. This simultaneously creates a low-threshold nature to the task. It should also be borne in mind that, in addition to the short time available, we rarely have large studios or richly equipped studios available in the consulting situation. As a result, we are basically "playing" a studio setting, a theater production, a studio, a TV spot, or a performance company. We are not work-creating artists in these moments, but people playing artists. It is serious play that does not tolerate casualness and inspires for that very reason. We cultivate the play in view of the actual art scene, and that is pleasurable and exciting without turning into a comedy. It is a work-creating play that can produce serious works that are sometimes even shown publicly.

5.4 Talk is silver; action is gold

In counseling, therapy, supervision, and coaching, the focus is on talking. And that certainly makes sense. However, it is striking that our experience, especially in counseling, supervision, and coaching situations, shows that a situation will most certainly only change for the better when the client takes action—specifically, when he tries something new in his everyday life and behaves differently. To put it in a nutshell, we could say that the most important task of the professional person is to get clients to act, —that is, to support them in trying out new behaviors.

This is plausible in many respects. Those who do something new or different in their everyday life cannot avoid having new experiences. They experience the effects of this action on themselves and others. They receive feedback. Above all, clients experience that even a feared failure, if it occurs, or the expected negative reaction of those involved does not "devastate" them. They learn that even negative results and consequences can be overcome so that it is not at all rare that they ultimately emerge strengthened from the situation in question. In this way, concrete action encourages and reinforces new action and enables clients to move from the position of victim to that of a doer and agent.

For art, acting is trivial in the sense that there is no art without action. Thus, there is also no Intermodal Decentering without action. This taking action does not happen because of the problem or its solution. It happens towards the art. The effect of artistic action is also trivial: there is something, or there is nothing. This effect is immediately detectable and cannot be explained away. Every person who gets involved in the artistic process will come to this "something," because the artistic work has a tendency to self-organization.

In this sense, artistic or playful activity proves to be a kind of sanctuary in which exploration can take place. Art and play not only enable but even force action, action that always leads to the goal.

This shows the importance of the decentering phase within a counseling session from a new perspective. In addition, decentering also proves to be a training ground in which action is practiced in a quasi-testing and, at the same time, binding manner. The effect of this action is clear, immediately apparent, and can be sensorially experienced. This may be one of the reasons why almost all clients, after a session with decentering, are spontaneously or by prompting ready to try something new in their everyday life in a very concrete way.

6

Metadiscourse on the Method and Its Effect

In Chapter 8, we will present in detail the roots of our methodical approach and the traditions of thought from which they stem. Already in Chapter 4, we have repeatedly come back to general observations and basic considerations in describing the details of our working method, while Chapter 5 refers to our fundamental understanding of language, art, and play.

The point of the following metadiscourse is not to repeat or anticipate these considerations. Rather, the first section summarizes our specific focus of attention while working with clients. We then describe the effects of our approach that we have observed so far in individual sessions and as we continue to work with clients. In other words, we reflect on the results, efficiency, and sustainability of Intermodal Decentering.

The last and most extensive section is devoted to the theoretical embedding of our methods. There, we go into detail about the concept of self-organization that has emerged within systems theory, as described by Kriz (e.g., 2006), Tschacher (2004), Haken and Schiepek (2006), and others. Through the experiments, research results, and theoretical considerations on self-organization, we believe it is easy to follow what is going on in a counseling or therapy session during a decentering phase and how the sometimes astonishingly positive effects can be explained.

In drawing on considerations of self-organization for the theoretical explanation of the power of action, the methodological approach of Intermodal Decentering presented here, we join a growing stream of scientific research and theory building to understand complex processes in nature and society. With the substitution model formulated here for the first time and the perspective of salutogenesis, we then move back into our own domain. These are additional attempts to make the effect of our methodological approach plausible.

6.1 Focus of attention

Phenomenological access

The prevailing mindset among professionals in the fields of therapy and counseling, even in the early years of the third millennium, has an orientation that we call structuralist. What is observed is understood as part of or indicative of a larger structured context. What is important is not so much how something shows up but what lies behind it. What is observed points to something more fundamental, more profound, or higher, and that is what is understood as central. Associated with this, for many professionals, is a particular fear of the impermanence, fleetingness, or seductiveness of the obvious.

A distinctively structuralist attitude understands what someone encounters as a symptom—that is, a sign or indication of a cause. Only the cause or causes have a binding quality of reality. The way something shows itself is suspected of being merely illusory.

Staying on the surface

In our work, we follow a different tradition, which has also found a home in art and solution orientation. In the practical process, we try to stay on the surface of what is designed and expressed. We call this approach "phenomenological" but without wanting to follow, for example, the various reductions of the founder of the corresponding philosophical direction (Husserl, 1952).

Phenomenology, the doctrine of appearances, of how something shows itself, wants to orient itself to the things themselves. It is interested in the actuality of the content under consideration and is equally concerned with the detailed description of the individual case. In doing so, it is aware of the fact that a person cannot keep in view the totality of all possible perspectives on a specific thing at any concrete moment.

To us, this phenomenological attitude towards what one encounters is essential. It requires, among other things, broad attention to everything soulful and a form of abstinence that shows itself in the effort to refrain from hasty evaluations, criticism, interpretations, theoretical interpretations, and the like.

This is why we speak of staying "on the surface," both in conversation with the client and in contact with his artistic work or playful activity. In other words, with this style that we cultivate, we avoid hastily reducing what shows itself to us to any categories.

From the point of view of shaping the relationship, such an attitude requires openness and a pronounced presence. It requires keeping an eye on the wholeness of the situation while appreciating the detail.

Furthermore, our focus of attention requires careful attention to language or expression. We take the other person "at their word." This means that we take the interlocutor seriously in her mode of expression, pay attention to unusual word choices, and possibly continue to use these expressions as a shared code.

The artistic work as "the third"

This basic attitude towards what we encounter is also reflected in the way we deal with the artistic work. Concrete work is verbally acquired by each person in a very different way. The encounter with the artistic work corresponds to the encounter with a counterpart, which develops, shows itself to the viewer in different ways, and holds surprises, thus possessing, so to speak, characteristics of a living counterpart. Of course, the people speak the words themselves. The work, however, puts them into their mouths.

A conversation between consultant and client would undoubtedly take a different course without the presence of the artistic work. At times, the conversation revolves strongly around the "third party in the alliance," around the "guest who has arrived," around whom both are striving. This third party is to be taken seriously in its unpredictability. We are called upon to confront what has "arrived" there, what shows itself.

The temptation is great to quickly reduce the challenging strangeness of the third to familiar patterns of interpretation, whereby one would remain in the familiar. Aesthetic analysis, which occupies an important place in this approach, does the opposite. It deals not only with the details of the work but also with its process of creation. It does this in descriptive language that is as concrete and detailed as possible. Client and guide walk around the work, for example, so that the diversity of perspectives is brought out. The words used, questions asked, and statements made highlight this diversity. It is the differences in perception that allow the work to show itself in its uniqueness. And thus, the ground is prepared for surprises.

However, this does not mean that we are not aware of our influence on what we observe. As will be explained in more detail in Section 8.3, we stand on the ground of social constructivism (Gergen, 2002) and therefore also understand a concrete observation as a joint construction of the participants. In our understanding, it is ultimately not possible to arrive at "the things themselves." Thus, strictly speaking, it is not even possible to merely "stay on the surface" when describing. But we can make an effort to do so. And we can do this in awareness of the manifold influences of an individual, situational, social, and cultural nature.

The effort to stay on the surface also does not mean that we ignore (behavioral) patterns. Even if every statement and every action is something unique, it can be beneficial to pay attention to regularities or patterns. Confronting a client with an observed pattern is like a change of perspective. It broadens the client's view and can be enriching and stimulating not only for understanding but also for future behavior. It is important to us that each observed pattern, although it represents a more abstract statement compared to a simple description of behavior, does not represent a truth of any higher order. And both remain constructions.

The phenomenological approach also has a strong influence on our approach to language, which we turn to in the following section.

Focus on language and content

Even though it is, of course, the client who determines the content with his concerns, the facilitator sets important accents within the process structure described in Chapter 4 through the nature of her questions.

In addition, the phenomenological approach determines the way something is put into language throughout all phases of the conversation. We focus on concrete, descriptive language that seeks to avoid abstractions and generalizations as much as possible. Adjectives and verbs are preferred over nouns. It is thus a matter of a verbal style instead of a nominal style. This is much more difficult in German than in English and represents a real challenge for some people.

Through the nature and phrasing of her questions and the way the counselor puts her observations into words, her style of speaking is brought home to the clients. With many clients, it can be observed over several sessions that the counselor's narrative style is gradually adopted. The consultant's approach thus has the effect of an indirect training program.

In terms of content, the focus is on the present or the immediate past and aspired futures. The former has our approach in common with all approaches of humanistic psychology. The latter is explained by the importance we attach to concretely formulated goals or imaginations of desired futures. "Good futures" described concretely in words have a positive pull effect and can, for example, develop a robust motivating force together with an appropriate artistic representation or a metaphor they have found themselves.

The temporal focus of attention described above must not be applied restrictively. Even things that happened long ago can become important in a phase of work with a client. In such situations, however, we strive also to work out the strengthening aspects of these usually stressful experiences and to establish a connection to the present.

6.2 Effects and sustainability

Effects in the first conversation phase

The effects described below have been observed in decentering work that started with a conversation phase according to the solution-oriented tradition.

This means that the phase preceding the decentering was not limited to the description of problems and difficulties. In addition, goals and "good results" were discussed, and exceptions to the problem state were talked about.

During the first phase of the discussion, it is always noticeable that people often laugh despite the seriousness of the situation described. There is a palpable sense of relief when the solution-oriented questions shed new light on something that had previously gone unnoticed. The mood seems to clear when a new perspective brings resources to light and, after further questions ("What else?"), previously unnoticed things become visible. There are many initial phases of conversation where surprises of this kind cause amazement.

Sometimes it happens in this phase of the conversation that the original problem relaxes, and something more fundamental comes to the fore. By expanding to "what is also present," the view opens up for personal qualities and new perspectives on the situation. This changes the basic attitude to one that physically and mentally allows a kind of alertness or even perplexity, and thus opens the gates to a committed curiosity. This state is a good prerequisite for decentering.

When clients experience these kinds of questions for the first time in the first phase, they are amazed at themselves and the resources they discover in connection with the problem. For example, if the counselor inquires about the circumstance that makes the issue most problematic, something amazing is often mentioned. Some clients quite excitedly begin to fight for their view of the problem. As a result, they have already stepped out of a victim attitude or suffering mood and are motivated to fight. Indirectly, they also show that they take possible other views seriously. In this case, asking what is important to the client in the context of the problem prepares the way for finding a solution. Some clients demand a clear appreciation of their suffering.

Effects in the decentering phase

This change of mood, the related sense of wonder, the readiness for surprises, and the alert, curious engagement that allows for amazement form the ideal condition for the challenge of a decentering play or artistic work. In this sense, the solution-oriented conversation in the first phase is a condition for the success of decentering.

The nature of the counselor's and client's presence in decentering manifests itself differently than in conversation. This is mainly because it is action-oriented and thus also involves the body. The alert curiosity and the committed desire for discovery express themselves here in action as eagerness and ambition. Both are driving moments of a creative power that is completely immersed in doing. The usual tendency to reflect is often put aside as a matter of course, and the tendency to interpret gives way to the reporting of experiences and the amazement at the work or play that has been created.

Effects during harvesting

The phase of harvesting shows itself as a speculative and associative space of conversation. Harvesting has to do with gathering what has ripened. The word "harvest" seems to us to be a helpful metaphor for this stage of the conversation because it also indicates that nothing can be forced here and that it is only a matter of selecting and bringing together what is significant at the moment.

During this phase of the conversation, the counselor often hears amazing verbal formulations, occasionally in poetic form, sometimes actual sentences of words of wisdom. "What's at hand now can go in very different directions, but I have to provide the impetus." "It's about both: the square and the round." "It's about including something from the gray area here and there." "It's like an eagle: flying freely over the stuff!"

If the counselor were to articulate such phrases as feedback or tips in the first phase of the conversation, she would probably often be met with skepticism, and the effect of the statement would fizzle out. However, since the sentences are formulated by the clients themselves, as explained in Section 4.8, they take on a completely different significance. This is because they are interpreted and concretized by the person himself.

One could describe the atmosphere in the phase of harvest as very open and the language as "winged." This atmosphere of openness makes one receptive to the world, to what is present right now. Many of the clients' sentences are ambiguous in their poetic style. Yet the experience that led to the statements is still present. In the subsequent concretization, this results in a large yield of possible meanings and inferences. This, in turn, leaves clients free to choose carefully, provided the counselor remains true to the premise that clients are experts on what is important at the moment and need only encouraging support in working out appropriate solutions.

Effects after the session is concluded

A successful decentering with a reasonably rich harvest usually leaves a thoughtful or stimulated client. The process with the elaborated aesthetic analysis and the self-found possible references to their own situation makes them become deeply involved. Very often, the clients also become curious about the effects of the outlined next steps.

It is astonishing how rarely, at the conclusion of a session with decentering, concerns or doubts are expressed about the feasibility of the planned further course of action. It was mentioned earlier (Section 4.9) that artistic activity can be understood metaphorically as "soul nourishment." If the focus of a decentering is predominantly on coping with an unfamiliar task that requires an aesthetic solution within a short time, the positive coping experience is more likely to be in the foreground. In a playful form of decentering, on the other hand, in addition to being stimulated, something like the "lightness of being" is often experienced. In any case, clients do feel a sense of well-being or, at the very least, a sense of being invigorated. The factor of self-efficacy often mentioned in recent literature and the confidence that something will change in a positive sense are likely to be significantly increased by our approach.

As described in Chapter 4, the facilitator is responsible for ensuring that the artistic or playful activity comes to a good end. The work must flourish to the point where it somehow appeals and begins to be liked. And it must be appropriately appreciated. This is likely to be one of the basic conditions for the client to feel highly affirmed and secure immediately after decentering and thus able to turn to new, unfamiliar, and undiscovered things. This affirmation is sometimes explicitly expressed: "I am already surprised that I started with this task just like that. And I have to say: I still like it!"

Reassurance can also refer to something you've always known and been aware of but often didn't really trust: "It works if I do not think too much and do not let myself be pressured. Actually, I've known that for a long time." This client's body language confirmed and completed this statement: she sat smiling mischievously and seemed like "an inside-out glove" compared to the beginning of the session.

Occasionally, the immediate impact of decentering work goes far beyond simple affirmation.

> In a demonstration session within a coaching training, Dora undergoes Intermodal Decentering, which, based on the coach's instructions, takes her from a small installation to a haiku (simple verse form) to a melodious expression. Dora ends with a long sustained, radiantly sung note. For a brief moment, the room is silent. All present are touched. In the post-session evaluation, Dora speaks of an "exhilarating

experience": "That long sound, the power of the place where I was standing...having that image (installation) in front of me." Half a year later, this experience is still very vivid and present for her.

In a similar mood, almost like in a slight trance, E. (see Section 4.8.) left the session after decentering.

In all situations in which the client feels stimulated or affected in a particular way after the decentering work—and this happens in the great majority—it seems to us useful, in order to continue this good state at the end of the session, to build a kind of bridge into everyday life (see Section 4.9). The feedback from the clients in the following session shows that such assistance can usually be put to good use.

Observations and reflections on sustainability

The immediate results of the decentering work are, on the one hand, sensorial experiences and, on the other hand, "second-degree solutions" put into language—that is, basic, sometimes metaphorical statements about the direction of the solution. Presumably, this mixture helps the experiences and considerations to stick amazingly well. So that concrete steps in the desired direction can be envisaged, it is usually useful to sketch them out together in the conversation with the help of the facilitator.

If, for example, an observation task is also given to take home, we often hear statements about the decentering experience in the next session, even after an interruption of several weeks, such as: "...has always accompanied me," "...was remembered as a happy experience," "...was in special situations like a yardstick for what is actually important to me."

"THE WAY I STAND IN LIFE"

For the head of a major restaurant chain, the idea of taking part in personal coaching would have been "unthinkable" just three years ago. That is how he expresses himself in the evaluation session that concludes the eight agreed meetings.

F. has worked his way up through discipline, skill, and drive from humble beginnings to his present managerial position, where about 100 managers report to him. Over the years, he acquired several procedures that proved to be effective and time-saving. They have now "become second nature" to him. For some time now, however, he has reached his limits.

This is most noticeable and nerve-wracking when dealing with one of his stepsons. But he also encounters the first difficulties in his own business. Based on the recommendation of a businessman in his circle of acquaintances, he signs up for personal coaching.

Being used to getting things done quickly and expeditiously, F. is pleased that the coaching sessions are also goal-oriented and concrete. In the counseling sessions, however, the counselor also tries to address fundamental aspects, something that is only possible in rudimentary form. Only the single decentering carried out in the fourth session provides the decisive impetus to do so.

F. is instructed to bring a creative task, which is entirely unfamiliar to him, under a certain amount of time pressure to a good end. He is relieved and surprised that he succeeds in doing so and that he also likes the resulting work. His insights in the harvesting phase emphasize the positive aspects of the attitude underlying F.'s behaviors which elsewhere provoke irritation in a number of places. At the same time, on a metaphorical level, possibilities for opening up and making this attitude more flexible are revealed. The coach, therefore, gives another designing task for the time before the next session, which includes possible expansions. F. dedicates himself to this task with care and perseverance.

The subsequent discussion of the "homework" and the further conversations show that F. is becoming increasingly aware that, in addition to pending behavioral changes in certain situations, "the way I stand in life" is up for debate. He confronts this issue. The coaching can be concluded after eight sessions, as planned.

In the closing session, F. reports various successes and actual highlights on different levels and repeatedly emphasizes that he has become "much more aware" of himself. He does not have the impression that "the job is done." He is "on the way." Visible steps had been taken, about which he had already received positive feedback from outsiders.

From the coach's point of view, a general movement has been set in motion. F. approaches himself and others with a broader and more tolerant mindfulness.

Decentering provides impetus

The example shows in a prototypical way that decentering alone is usually not enough. Especially not when fundamental attitudes and long-standing behavior patterns are at play. Here it is necessary to stimulate, support, and consolidate the process of clarification or change by working on concrete situations, by a kind of attention training with regard to one's resources and strengths, by support, by sensitization, by homework, and suggestions for experiments and much more. An initial decentering usually provides important impulses in this process, and it conveys sensorial experiences that can be used by the client as a kind of anchor in the later course. Further decentering within such a process helps to clarify further, supports concrete steps, and draws attention to additional dimensions that need to be considered.

Decentering enables sustainable conflict resolution

This kind of process can be observed in therapies and counseling, but also in many coaching sessions. In supervision sessions, on the other hand, as well as in certain counseling situations, it happens again and again that after a single session with decentering, a specific problem is worked through to such an extent that it can subsequently be handled by the client herself without significant support. This is the rule rather than the exception, even in the case of professional conflict situations of female newcomers to the profession. Therefore, unless it is a training situation where a certain number of supervision sessions is mandatory, such counseling can often be successfully completed after only three or four sessions. If these clients wish to continue in counseling, a change in the subject matter can usually be observed. The focus is then no longer on concrete problems or conflict situations from everyday work, but the conversation begins to turn to questions of how to shape one's life and quality of life.

Unexpected concrete steps of the clients

If one observes somewhat more systematically the concrete steps that clients take to change their situation after a session with decentering, one finds that it is not at all uncommon for these to be steps that were not outlined at all in the session. They are indeed quite consistent with the general direction that emerged in the "second-degree solutions." The concrete execution, however, is often unexpected for the consultant. Sometimes concrete measures have obviously become unnecessary because the situation changed as if by itself in the desired direction. Alternatively, the client has thought of something simpler, occasionally something "crazier" to do. Now and then, the client decides to make a change in another area of life first, which also defuses the situation in the problem area.

Such observations remind the counselor to be humble. For us, they are a sign of the power of self-organization—of the self-healing power—of the person system or the social systems involved. It is true that considerations for concrete steps worked out in the counseling session can be quite valuable and are also taken up by the client. But more importantly, they seem to be the appreciative, supportive, curious, surprising, creative, and pleasurable moments of the decentering work.

Sustainable long-term effects

The long-term effects of working with decentering observed so far are promising. Our observations now span six to ten years. The change steps stimulated and supported by decentering seem to be sustainable and can be integrated into the clients' corresponding life concepts, which often also experience changes. When inquiring after one or two years, a single decentering experience is mentioned only very rarely. More often, however, one hears the statement that the sessions "where we did something else" were particularly valuable (meaning: did something other than just talk).

It should be critically noted that in everyday practice, the effect of decentering cannot be distinguished from the effect of the entire counseling or therapy process. From our point of view, the professional is responsible for two things: he must enable the client to have a sensorial experience in the decentering activity, and he must design the part of language in such a way that language remains entirely "on the surface" in the decentering phase, and resource-oriented descriptions are cultivated in the other phases. As of the writing of this chapter, no systematic studies have been conducted on the impact of decentering work. In addition, it must be noted that there are no severe mental disorders among the clientele observed.

Decenterings with no discernible effects?

Are there decenterings without recognizable effects on the clients or the counseling or therapeutic process? In principle, this must be expected. In reality, however, it has been observed very rarely up to now.

> A highly intelligent young academic with strongly rationalizing speaking behavior and tremendous self-doubt only partially gets involved in the task of decentering and restricts himself to a conventional solution. Nevertheless, some interesting associations arise in the "harvest," but their concretization in everyday life quickly peters out.

This example gives a first indication of the limitations of the application of Intermodal Decentering. We will discuss this in more detail in Section 7.2.

6.3 Theoretical thoughts on the effectiveness

In Chapter 8, we will describe in detail the roots and traditions of thought that have inspired the development of our approach. This is a specific conception of art, based on phenomenology, in which the sensorial aspect of artistic activity and the aesthetic commitment are specifically emphasized. Furthermore, it is the resource-oriented approach to conversation, which emphasizes the client's maturity with its system-theoretical, humanistic, and contructivistic roots.

In Chapter 3, reference was made to theory groups that are close to our thinking. Among others, Watzlawick's concept of "more of the same" (e.g., Watzlawick *et al.*, 1969) was mentioned there, pointing out that supposed solutions to conflicts often exacerbate the problem. Anything that leads away from "more of the same" is likely to be potentially helpful. Furthermore, there were considerations about creativity because it is characterized definitionally by the fact that a new approach is taken in a known situation or that an old solution is surprisingly applied in a new situation. Art realizes creativity. The reflections on imagination proved that greater scope is available when the imaginative is accentuated. Likewise, certain game theories indicate the same for the field of action. Theories of Conflict finally point out that one has to step out of the field of conflict with advantage if solutions are to be found. This principle applies in summary to all theoretical approaches referred to in this chapter.

In this last main section of the metadiscourse on our approach and its effects, we address three theoretical approaches that frame, from different perspectives, the processes that take place in Intermodal Decentering. They are close to our own thinking and can offer alternative explanations for the observed effects. These are the synergetics—respectively, the self-organization theories, the substitution model designed by Knill, and the perspective of salutogenesis.

Systemic approach, self-organization, synergetics

Systems theory is a cornerstone of our thinking. It directs the view to the whole of a situation and tries to grasp volatile processes as well as more persistent structures (patterns) in the complexity of the given.

Inspired mainly by the work of Jürgen Kriz (e.g., 1997a, 1997b, 2002), we have increasingly dealt with the phenomenon of self-organization in the last decade. In doing so, we have come across the ideas of synergetics, which was founded by Hermann Haken's (e.g., 1995) theoretical description of the phenomena observed in laser beams.

Synergetics explains the formation and self-organization of patterns and structures in open systems that exist far from thermodynamic equilibrium. It is now widely supported not only in the natural sciences (physics, chemistry, biology) but also in mathematics, sociology, and psychology, and thus corresponds to our interdisciplinary approach. The synergetic approach fascinates us because it attempts to map complexity without premature reduction.

Summarized and popularized in an almost inadmissible way, it involves the following.

The problem with order

Human life appears in the tension between chaos and constricting order. Chaos alone is deadly. Without order, life is inconceivable. However, every order means at the same time potentially a massive restriction of degrees of freedom or—formulated from another perspective—a reduction of complexity. The latter is what makes order(s) so attractive to humans. Such orders were described within psychology a long time ago—for instance, by Piaget (e.g., 1937) as schemata or by Metzger (e.g., 1962) and other Gestalt theorists as Gestalt laws. Riedl (after Kriz, 1997a) speaks of innate patterns of complexity reduction, which would have proved to be capable of survival in the course of evolution.

Kriz (2004) has pointed out that parallel to complexity reduction, a completion dynamic can often be observed. The human cognitive system completes weakly recognizable orders into an overall picture (e.g., image recognition of the human face).

Accordingly, order is created by the reduction of complexity. However, if we reduce everything to a few familiar categories, we miss the uniqueness of experiences. Individuals, collectives, and societies in the Western world seem to tend towards an excess of order. While this initially creates a certain sense of security, it can result in stress, problems, conflicts, and even mental and physical illness in the long run.

The conclusion from this described sequence seems obvious: creativity in acting and thinking, the joy and enjoyment of unique experiences, and flexibility in encountering new situations—all this presupposes a certain openness to the chaotic. Or vice versa: in consulting situations, we usually deal with an excess of order in our clients. To put it more precisely, people who seek counseling or therapy find themselves in a disturbed balance between the poles of chaos and congealed order.

How change happens

Systems theory has shown that systems tend to remain in dynamic equilibrium once it has been found. In technical language, one speaks of persistence in an "attractor" (see below). This behavior has the great advantage that minor fluctuations in environmental conditions can always be compensated for. A continuous change in these conditions, however—for example, a continued increase in time pressure at the workplace or a person's steadily aging body— can permanently alter the equilibrium. The pattern of behavior that may have worked well to very well for a long time becomes increasingly inappropriate. The (old) order becomes a problem (see the above example of F.: "The way I stand in life" in Section 6.2). Through experiments in non-human systems, for example, in the field of physics and chemistry, a "critical slowdown" could be observed. This means that the adaptability of the system to the old equilibrium (the old attractor) is slowed down in a striking way.

If the change in environmental conditions, known in technical language as control parameters, continues, the system enters a state of unstable equilibrium, where even small fluctuations are enough to nudge it on the path to a new attractor—that is, a new equilibrium.

Such a reorganization never occurs in a linear fashion but rather in leaps and bounds, often unexpectedly and suddenly. It can be experienced as a very dramatic change. Very many reorganizations, however, are unspectacular, and one often notices them only in retrospect. In everyday language, one speaks of having "learned something." However, when it comes to actual life patterns, such learning processes can never completely eliminate previously developed states of order. In stressful situations, the old pattern can be reactivated: We speak of a "relapse" (Haken and Schiepek, 2006).

Self-organization

The ability of systems to maintain their structure even under changing environmental conditions and—in the case of further environmental changes— to change this structure themselves without direct external influence can be understood as self-organization. Accordingly, the term "self-organization" includes simple equilibrium processes, which are maintained with control loop structures (feedbacks), as well as actual structural changes, which can be described with the word "learning." In the literature, "self-organization" is used as a generic term for expressions such as "self-repairing system," "self-generating system," or "learning system."

The term was first used in the natural sciences to distinguish the independent emergence of ordered structures from an externally determined order.

For the understanding of self-organization processes, the concept of the attractor plays an important role. The attractor is a mathematically defined phenomenon—more precisely, an abstract mathematical principle. Within systemic thinking, one speaks of an ordered dynamic structure, which has a remarkable resistance to perturbations (e.g., a candle flame). Attractors contribute massively to the reduction of complexity in everyday life.

We could not function without them. However, the longer and stronger such an attractor works, the more ingrained a pattern is and the greater the danger that it will not be adaptable enough to new requirements. The attractor then becomes a problem itself.

In human systems, interaction systems but also patterns of meaning interpretation ("meaning attractors"; Kriz, 1997b) are in the foreground. Interaction dynamics, as well as sense-making and interpretation dynamics, can be understood as attracting processes. Imagination and fantasy are also significant attracting forces. This is one of the reasons why desirable future states can develop great forces for ordering life processes.

The question of how far and in what way external conditions can influence the mental system is of great importance for the understanding of the processes in the counseling situation. After all, counseling itself represents a form of external influence. It seems to be certain that the connection between the change of external conditions and the change of a system is not linear—that is, small causes can have a big effect.

Similarly, observable changes in humans cannot be attributed solely to external influences. On the contrary, decades ago, studies of other, relatively simple, living systems—for example, the cell (cf. Maturana and Varela, 1987), showed that a direct influence on the processes inside the system is not possible at all. Transferred to the counseling situation, this means that the possibility of a direct content-related counseling influence ("instructive interaction") into a person's mental system is ruled out according to our current understanding.

With constant changes in the external conditions, which aim in the same direction, the affected system changes discontinuously. The ongoing consultative unsettling of ingrained, limiting beliefs, for example, which may seem ineffective for an extended period, may suddenly manifest success.

The transition from one dynamic structure to another

Establishing order in a disorderly situation is usually done unobtrusively. Ambiguous signals or insufficient information are evaluated, supplemented, and usually enriched with material from memory. All this happens in a self-evident way quickly, often erratically. The well-known ambiguous, tilting figures from perception theory are an impressive example of this.

The situation becomes somewhat different when, for example, an existing behavior pattern that is no longer adequate is transformed into a new one. This is much more difficult for most of us. We often hesitate, even if the insight of the necessity of such a change has been there for a long time. Old orders—that is, existing attractors—often have great persistence. And this is then sometimes the starting point for which the professional competence of a counselor is called upon.

It must be assumed that the transition from an old order to a new one is always associated with a destabilized state. This means that without disturbing experiences, without more or less gentle questioning, without contradiction, little or nothing happens. At the same time, counselors and clients must be prepared for this period of instability. If the instability becomes too great, there is a danger of destructive or otherwise dysfunctional "solutions."

In such a phase of transition, the counseling process itself can provide support. A certain degree of ego strength in the client, the activation of resources, experiences of control as well as experiences of self-efficacy are further important factors for critical transitions to be endured and mastered in a good way.

The critical slowdown observed in the synergy experiments, which draws attention to the increasing destabilization of the system equilibrium (the old attractor), is also likely to be important in terms of counseling. It could be the confusion often observed when something new becomes forebodingly visible to clients.

What does all this mean for counseling?

The aim is to create conditions for the self-organization process that are experienced as useful by the client and his environment. This means that the counselor is expected not so much to be competent in analyzing the content of a problem or existing pattern but to be competent in shaping the process of change.

As already emphasized several times, a direct influence on the content from the outside is not possible. What is possible, however, are methods of context control, which in a favorable case "enable the system to organize itself and to adopt a less suffering, healthier attractor" (Strunk and Schiepek, 2006, p.271). The content of the new attractor cannot be predetermined. To ensure that it is not left entirely to chance, it is vital to work on positive visions of the future beforehand. Nor can the appearance of the new be fixed precisely in time. Especially in psychotherapeutic settings, but also in other entrenched problem situations, it would be helpful to identify the time of transition early on. At these times, systems are susceptible and open to disruption so that appropriate interventions can achieve a high degree of effectiveness. In very elaborate time series analyses, a research group around the Munich psychologist Günter Schiepek tries to identify such input-sensitive phases (e.g., Schiepek *et al.*, 2005).

Within a counseling process, the task of the professional is, among other things, to "de-automate" what has been taken for granted so far, as expressed in the attractor that is in the foreground (Kriz, 2002). In other words, it is a matter of stepping out of the emergency or the narrowness of a previous focus and introducing and adopting new perspectives. These are not "more correct" new perspectives, but different ones, and, if possible, a variety of others, enriching the understanding of the situation. If the counselor ensures that such multi-perspectivity is endurable, this can be experienced and understood as both energizing and cognitively disorienting. Both contribute to facilitating the seeking out of a new attractor.

How is the decentering phase to be understood from this perspective?

The introduction of a phase of decentering and the use of artistic and playful means take the client out of his everyday world. We speak of the transition from an everyday to an alternative reality. This can be understood as stepping out of the stream of the self-evident and distancing oneself from it. With the attitude cultivated towards the client, the latter becomes much more of a creator, a "doer" of his own life, and a possible role of victim recedes into the background.

In the harvesting phase, clients are asked to see things in a completely different, more playful way for once—that is, to see connections where there are hardly any connections from everyday logic. One can understand this with Kriz as "de-automating the self-evident." In harvesting, fixed connections and convictions become, on a trial basis, ambiguous, vague, for the time being completely undetermined and yet somehow attractive possibilities and hypotheses.

In the harvesting phase, the complexity of the interpretation is significantly increased. This further stabilizes the situation and, at the same time, "energizes" it through the many new pieces of information. Kriz (2007) points out that the increase of energy in physical systems corresponds to the enrichment of information in communicative, meaning-generating systems. Both accelerate the process in the area of a "phase transition," as such qualitative changes of state are called in the literature. Since it must be assumed in principle that, typically, in an attractor landscape, numerous alternatives are available in times of phase transitions, the chance is high that one of them will come into play.

The openness of the conversation in this phase, the variety of hypotheses developed during the harvesting, the observation tasks often suggested after a session, the trial exploration of new behaviors, the resource-oriented atmosphere during the conversations, and more are precautions to ensure that the client neither hastily sticks to a particular scenario nor remains in an indecisive state for a longer period of time.

The artistic process as a self-organizing experience

Every artistic work arises from chaos. The white canvas, the silence, the empty space, and the blank page correspond in their emptiness or fullness to chaotic states. They are often described as frightening even by creative people. Every creative action within this chaos has an ordering character.

Only when the work emerges as something surprising, which cannot be predicted exactly, is it generally considered an artistic work. Accordingly, this process is not about mapping, implementing, or even enforcing a pre-planned order. But rules, methods, or a course of action can be prescribed. However, there must still be so much chaos that surprising developments can arise.

In the artistic process, the result of acts of art is enrichment. Thus a dynamic of attraction develops, and phase transitions become possible, making the work appear more and more. There are rhythmic, structural, symmetrical, geometric, motivic, figurative, and similar attractors that enable certain designs in one direction or another. The work organizes itself, so to speak, and the shapers serve or follow what is showing or "revealing itself" until the phenomenon occurs of the shaper saying, "It's done." Subsequently, the process can be traced; it is not recognizable in advance. Kriz (2002) understands this attracting dynamic, which pulls, so to speak, into the future of the work, as teleological.

This phenomenon applies to decentering in general. We consider below what influence this richness in experiencing the self-organization of a work can have on the self-organization process of solutions.

The inclusion of the work in the consulting system

Work, client, and therapist are in a kind of three-way confrontation. They are part of a system and interact in a second-order cybernetics (Kriz, 1997a, p.56). As the interventions in artistic design are probed exploratorily for their effect, the possibilities enrich themselves tangibly, and, with them, the fields of meaning and significance needed for solutions. This enrichment is always sensorially perceptible, palpable, tangible, and thus also verbally accessible and reflectable for all. Since, during decentering, the usual orders of thought from the everyday context subside, surprising new areas of meaning and significance can appear on all levels.

Such areas concern, for example:

- The differentiation and expansion of perception through the surprising appearance of the surface of the work. This illustrates the differentiation and expansion of perception in everyday life.
- The reflection on which interventions were effective in the work process. Unexpected possibilities for action are demonstrated.
- The richness of experience during the creative process. It can expand the emotional playing range.

This enrichment is further magnified by multiple perspectives from the different levels of observation that clients are invited to use during the aesthetic analysis of the work. This double enrichment through new fields of meaning and multiple perspectives is, as has already been shown, interesting from the point of view of systems theory since it favors a phase transition.

However, when enrichments primarily emphasize the problem-laden issue, they can potentially build an anxiety barrier. Since, in decentering, the problem-laden subject is not brought into the artistic process, and the challenge in decentering is primarily through artistic activity related to the self-organization of the work, this kind of double enrichment can be navigated.

The substitution model

If, as shown at the beginning, we consider decentering as a change analogous to the solution process, which in its play range expansion makes us "forget" the problem under consideration, then we could say somewhat casually that the initial concern is substituted by an alternative playful artistic concern with surprising solutions. With this model, which we call the "substitution model," we can provide a possible approach to clarification. We do this by showing in both processes of resolution—namely, within the concern and in addressing the decentering task—that the same categories of resolution experiences are possible, but each in a different way.

We preliminarily isolated six categories and examined them within the situation of confinement or lack (*Notenge*). We then examined whether aesthetic analysis can reveal changes in these categories in the decentering process. These categories are devoted to the following phenomena, and they show up in the concern as summarized here:

- **Phenomena of inability, of not being capable.** At the beginning of every counseling, there is an inability, the search for help.
- **Phenomena of lack of resources.** It is one of the basic assumptions of our concept that resources are hidden.
- **Phenomena of view and perspectives.** The perspective is narrow and one-sided; blind spots exist.
- **Phenomena of agency.** Lack of scope and the seemingly unsolvable paralyze agency.
- **Phenomena of language and communication.** The poor language, the rigid thinking process, the spinning in circles.
- **Phenomena in the body–mind continuum.** Irrational ways of thinking or acting, limited emotional competencies.

If we now pay attention to these categories in the aesthetic analysis and work out how these phenomena have changed in the work or play process, then the changes can be paraphrased as follows.

PHENOMENA OF INABILITY, NOT BEING CAPABLE, AND LACK OF RESOURCES ARE POSITIVELY CHANGED

The client has experienced the view of inability in the "I can't create" differently and, in addition, has mastered the situation with limited resources, provided that a coherent work has emerged. The success is rewarded by beauty, an "aha" experience, an aesthetic resonance.

PHENOMENA OF VIEW AND PERSPECTIVES ARE ENRICHED

Since the work in its creation and its presence always offers different perspectives of perception, a differentiation of perception and enrichment of views with the concrete of the work or, as we say, at the surface is possible. Effective perceptual enrichment naturally requires that the therapist also participates in this reflection on the surface of the work as an appreciative observer. In this context, the clients practice multi-perspective perception, which will facilitate adopting an additional point of view for everyday life.

PHENOMENA OF THE ABILITY TO ACT ARE EXPANDED

The action of going to work and coming out again is always part of the becoming of a work. The aesthetic process analysis is dedicated to the actions and measures, the successes and difficulties, and what helped to stay with it. Such actions and overcoming difficulties in artistic practice can give clues to actions in everyday life in the harvesting phase.

PHENOMENA OF LANGUAGE AND COMMUNICATION ARE ENRICHED

The language of the work can only be understood through itself—that is, metaphors, images, actions, movements, sounds, and words open to many possibilities of conversation—and cannot be pinned down to a single correct one. In the "studio," therefore, there is intense communication going on with and about the work and the related questions of technique, which expands the everyday language of conversation.

This enrichment of communication takes place on the surface of the work when we ask about differences in the experience of the studio phase and about surprises. Reflection on the work is also pleasantly distanced from the purely personal. The enrichment of the conversation related to the work and the design process in connection with a distancing from the purely personal leads to a more objective and expanded understanding of the everyday situation and to approaches to solutions during the harvesting.

PHENOMENA IN THE BODY–MIND CONTINUUM BECOME MORE PERMEABLE

Artistic expression belongs to humanity like language. However, it is a language of a different kind. Poetry, in its innovative use of words, becomes a "thinking of a different kind" (Fuchs, 2002, p.162). At the same time, in artistic activity, one is sensorially and physically engaged, even if this engagement varies in different art disciplines. In any case, all senses are always engaged in artistic activities. This happens as a matter of course and always in the context of what is revealed in the very act of creating. The experience of the body–soul engagement in decentering is also productive because it can be assigned not only to the ego but also to the work since the imaginary space of art (stage or canvas) allows for modes of action and possibilities that cannot necessarily be assigned to the creator.

They are, so to speak, exploratory actions without consequences. Being sensorially engaged and at the same time distancing the creator from the work enables the expansion of emotional competencies.

A perspective of salutogenesis

If artistic expression is considered as a human existential and not symptomatic of a pathological development, the turn to salutogenesis (Bengel *et al.*, 1998) and the importance of resources also belong to the theoretical basis. Since creative activity as an existential, with its surprising experiences, is related to dreaming and daydreaming, it belongs, like these, to the realm of what is called "soul." It could be metaphorically called "soul sustenance."

The experience justifies such a designation. Many clients fondly remember their work processes, and, not infrequently, the work of a group or team is set up at the place of work or performed again on a special occasion. The positive influence this can be expected to have on the corresponding group or team culture can be understood in the context of resilience, the ability to activate one's resources (Schiffer, 2001, p.11). Seen in this way, artistic activity is not only part of overcoming human suffering but just as much part of enabling social competence.

In decentering, one's strengths are mobilized in order to find one's way out of situations of distress, confinement, or lack. Schiffer says that "despite stress, those who can play with all their senses and then bring these bodily experiences of play into speech have good prospects of health" (2001, p.11). This view is close to the theory of salutogenesis. The medical sociologist Antonovsky created this term as an antithesis to pathogenesis. It can be translated as "health emergence." He points out that, according to Antonovsky, health is not a state but a process.

Schiffer (2001, p.49) also shows that the "affectu-sensomotor-" experiences (as experienced in play and artistic activity) are fundamental to mobilizing resilience. Below, using the same criteria as worked on in the substitution model, it will be shown how in decentering resilience and access to resources are made possible.

Symptom: Inability (I can't do it)

In the face of the problem, the symptom grows. If the counselor steps in to give solutions, it intensifies because it demonstrates the inability of one's searching. "It's so simple, see that's how you solve it!" In the artistic task, the symptom appears to be new vis-à-vis the task ("I am not gifted"), but within the decentering method, it is coped with by the client from his own resources, and this coping, when recognized, becomes significant in the harvesting phase.

Symptom: There is a lack of resources

In the face of the problem, the symptom is so strong that it blinds us to our resources.

In every artistic creation or play, the symptom is present in the limitations of resources (frame and material) because these limitations belong to the essence of play. At a distance from the problem, they are surprisingly mastered in playful, pleasurable challenge. This coping also becomes an existential experience available in the harvesting phase.

Symptom: Weakness to act

In view of the problem, this symptom increases in the hopelessness of the situation. In the artistic task, the symptom is initially present as inhibition but is soon overcome through the experimentation and trial and error present in the play and artistic activity with an open outcome.

Symptom: Cognitive rigidity and low impetus

Due to the problem, the symptom worsens as the cycle of despair continues with no resolution in sight.

In the artistic task, for the time being, a similar symptom appears in the tendency to want to solve the task rationally in a planning way. However, the physically and mentally heightened engagement of any artistic activity, far from the problem, soon becomes a fascination with surprises, so that this inhibiting tendency gives way to an engagement in self-forgetfulness. The harvest then begins in an enthusiastic mood, which is conducive to overcoming the problem.

In this context, the experience of crisis interventions in disaster areas can also be pointed out. These are the situations in which the mobilization of resilience is existential. It is reported that the use of cultural-artistic resources proves to be very helpful (Lahad, 1992).

7

The Application and Its Limits

7.1 Areas of application

Therapy

The method of Intermodal Decentering originated in the field of therapy. However, it was developed in detail and initially applied on a broader scale in the fields of supervision and coaching. Historically, this is partly due to the different framework conditions in the various professional fields.

The resource- and goal-oriented understanding of settings and roles in Intermodal Decentering was originally closer to the counseling profession than to the clinical profession. As stated in Chapter 8, in the field of expressive arts therapy, artistic expression is understood as a natural, culturally rooted, bodily sensorial phenomenon with strong imaginative content. The focus is on the sensorial. The reductionist reinterpretation or interpretation of the artistic work as an image of something "deeper," for example, in the sense of a psychodiagnosis, was not cultivated and rejected. Within the therapeutic setting, the positive effect of artistic activity was originally seen mainly in the cathartic effect and/or in finding meaning or in the phenomenological dialogue with the work. Today, in contrast, the aspect of enrichment and strengthening comes to the fore, together with the learning and coping effect and, above all, the support of self-organization—that is, the actualization of the self-healing forces. Thus, the turn towards a resource-oriented approach has occurred.

In the field of therapy, art-oriented work usually has to adjust to a more extended period of time, and in the clinical field, it often has to deal with severely impeded communication. This can interfere with adherence to the formal process presented. We must then settle in to work on the piece over several sessions, as may be the case in counseling, for example, when painting a picture. With ephemeral media, such as music, we then continue with what is still present in the next session. The disturbance may be so permeated by the symptomatic that we cannot step away entirely from the problematic, and we are required to undertake crisis intervention.

This may result in the artistic process temporarily fading into the background. In other words, during the artistic process, the therapist cannot only concentrate on the role of the studio director but must be prepared to deal directly with a disturbance of the relationship out of therapeutic responsibility. How this is done in concrete terms depends on the school of therapy that has helped to shape the intervention style of the particular therapist.

This means that such interventions should not lead to giving up the aesthetic responsibility for the emerging work as this would diminish the surprise and immediacy of the work process. In therapeutic use, therefore, one is challenged in two ways. On the one hand, clinical experience and therapeutic responsibility must always be ready in the sense of the art-analogical stance, and, at the same time, the emerging work should come to the fore through the interventions out of aesthetic responsibility (cf. Lempert, 2007, p.106).

There are similar deviations from the formal process in the therapeutic use of aesthetic analysis to the work or progress of the work (in processes over several sessions). The emotional component of artistic creation and the impact of the work on the client's mood often take precedence, so we must address them before discussing the process or the surface of the work. Contents and meanings (of the artwork) can be addressed and are often directly related to the clients suffering or problem. Lempert (2007, p.117) uses an exemplary case (dance as an artistic work) to illustrate the process of an aesthetic work reflection in therapy. He shows how, over the course of several sessions, an aesthetic responsibility towards the work is carried out in the aesthetic analysis of a work and how the client can be led away from the emotional to reflect on the work and the process repeatedly.

Even what we have described as "harvesting" (see Section 4.8) can be an important component of resource-based therapy, especially when working with goal-setting.

Even if the formal process of Intermodal Decentering is not always applied as such in therapy, the method and its derivation, as shown in Chapter 4, have brought an important aspect of effect into creative therapies. Paying attention to the content of the image or work as an important triangulation in the therapeutic relationship receives an additional essential extension through the analysis of the aesthetic reality of the creative process.

Intermodal Decentering thus means an alternative experience of the world that mobilizes resources and overcomes challenges in the concrete creation of the work in therapy.

Supervision and coaching

In contrast, the situation in the field of supervision and coaching is significantly different from that in the therapeutic context.

Here, clients expect insights into correlations that are difficult for them to understand or are looking for solutions in personally difficult or inherently complex professional and life situations. These clients do not feel sick or disabled at all. From their point of view, they are in a tricky situation from which they want to find their way out with the help of a professional. However, a simple explanation or tip usually does not help them because they have already tried various things themselves without success, and not even the advice of professional colleagues and friends has been of any use.

In a coaching or supervision situation, the aim is to open up new perspectives within a relatively short time, making use of the strengths and possibilities that lie within the client and his situation. The solution- and resource-oriented conversational approach already serves this purpose very well. The additional use of art- or play-oriented methods in the form of decentering adds another dimension.

Sometimes the introduction of a decentering phase is greeted with hesitation by the client when it is carried out for the first time and is perceived as a risk or a small adventure. However, if the established relationship was sufficiently sustainable and the phase was described as an "experiment," then, in our experience, everyone without exception has been able to get involved. Once it is experienced that what has been worked out in decentering opens up completely new perspectives and can be used beneficially, the client is more than willing to get involved in it again. Some are even slightly disappointed when later sessions do not include decentering.

Based on the starting point described above, both coaching and supervision situations have so far proven to be very suitable for Intermodal Decentering. However, here, too, certain preconditions must be taken into account.

That someone really gets involved in the artistic or playful activity in a decentering phase presupposes something like playful seriousness. This requires a protected framework. It is true that there are people—most often female—who like to engage in a "little excursion" within counseling.

However, they, too, need to be sure that the counselor is genuinely concerned about their issue and is doing everything possible not to embarrass the client. Most clients, however, are initially insecure, slightly anxious, or skeptical, and need the certainty that they will not be ridiculed in order to really get involved in what is usually a completely unexpected and often very unfamiliar activity. For one author (H.E.), this is one reason why he rarely performs decentering in an initial interview.

For example, some coaching clients have experienced experiments and surprising arrangements being used as a gimmick in leadership training.

If one wanted to use an artistic or playful decentering episode in this sense in this context—as a pleasant interruption of the conversation, for example, or as something "one could do for a change"—it would probably be worthless, if not counterproductive, for the continuing consulting process. We suspect that casualness in decentering activity is fatal for the result: engaging in an artistic activity requires a certain ease, but at the same time full presence. This is supported by curiosity and possibly also a little daring. But in no case can it tolerate casualness. In the case of a work that has been created only casually, the aesthetic analysis can become a farce, and the harvest is likely to be meager to meaningless.

However, some clients are not confident in artistic creation and, therefore—for example, in an installation task—are very quickly satisfied with a form once it has been found. In such a situation, the counselor's thoughtful, understanding guidance is necessary, which helps to pay more attention to and appreciate the aesthetic qualities of what has been created and, if necessary, to improve them in the form of reworking.

> K.V. has quickly finished his installation and sees no more possibilities to change his work. The counselor, therefore, sets him the task of selecting two objects from the room and placing them within the installation so that the aesthetic quality is fundamentally altered but remains appealing.

In this way, the resulting work can acquire a whole new artistic value in the eyes of its creator, which often astonishes the person concerned.

The evaluations of decentering in coaching and supervision situations have so far almost always proved valuable for the further progress of the counseling. Sometimes they were even the decisive turning point for finding a solution, especially when the problem involved quite personal aspects.

However, if the issue to be addressed approaches a technical or project consultation, decentering is not necessarily the appropriate method.

Working with groups

Clients who gather in groups around a concern or are specially assembled are found in therapy, education, counseling, and supervision. Small groups also gather around cultural needs, educational needs, and community concerns such as political concerns (e.g., setting up pedestrian zones), church concerns (e.g., the need for cohesion), or association concerns (e.g., conflict resolution).

Today, we also encounter more large groups with cultural concerns that come together primarily for "community work" and, in our case, "community art."

Even though teams are often a myth, there are differences between the group and the team on two levels, as we will see in the next section.

The loose structure of the group. The individual group members usually come together because of a specific interest, so they are primarily interest-based and hardly ever share their daily work routine for the sake of a common task. For this reason, a certain amount of time in each group meeting usually needs to be devoted to group formation and group culture.

The individual nature of the concern. Although a group may meet out of a common interest in case supervision or therapy, each group member brings a different case or concern. Even with educational needs, the educational process is different for participants. However, the individual learning process can gain from the shared group work.

When working with Intermodal Decentering in groups, care must be taken to ensure that the structure of the decentering phase corresponds to the concerns of the individual group members. In principle, three forms of guidance are suitable for this purpose:

For an individual concern (e.g., case supervision):

- **Individual work** (the personal situation is the focus): the group has observation tasks and gives feedback.
- **Protagonist work** (the concern is, e.g., the group member's client is the focus of concern): The whole group participates (one part can take over observation tasks). The artistic offer requires an ensemble structure with a special position taken by the person with the individual concern (cf. below).

For a common cause (e.g., educational assignment):

- The whole group works on an artwork or play, and individuals get their individual harvest from a shared aesthetic analysis.

The offer of art to groups should always be appropriate to the nature of the concern of the group member at the center. It is helpful if the resources of the group are fully utilized. In our work, we also refer to resources that have to do with art and the ability to play. These come into play not only in active participation in decentering but also in aesthetic analysis and harvesting, where involving the group can be very enriching.

The following considerations can help you make the best use of resources when choosing what to offer:

Individual work within a large group tends to become a classical demonstration and is to be avoided outside the training or lecture setting. Instead, consider dividing the group into an ensemble with protagonists, roles, and an audience with observational tasks.

In protagonist work, guidance can be gained from the tradition of the arts. Here are a few examples:

- In an ensemble dance performance, the protagonist may participate as a choreographer and then, as the work progresses, may dance in the company herself or take the part of the soloist. Such decisions often arise from the concern.
- In the case of a mural, she may take on the role of coordinator for the division of space.
- In an improvisation close to the jazz tradition, she may take on the role of arranger or the solo part.
- In theater, she may be the assistant director, or she may set the location, the scene, and the beginning of the action of the improvisation.

It should always be the decision of the protagonist—in the role of the arranger or choreographer—that is adopted in the various takes or versions. Fellow performers are then asked to what extent they can take over the instructions. In a sense, the protagonist receives art coaching and is at the center of the session.

In the case of **group concerns**, the classical ensemble form is observed; everyone is equally responsible for giving shape to the work. To avoid long discussions, it is advisable for the leadership to propose finding a decision through attempts at action, rather than forcing artistic solutions through discussion.

For cultural tasks, "community art" comes into play when working with communities and very large groups. It is based on the method of Intermodal Decentering and is primarily intended for use in settings where the group can be understood as a system that has a common concern (cf. Knill, 2007, p.165). This use may exist in the context of counseling or educational assignments. The system may be temporarily committed to collaboration, as in a training or project management assignment, or it may have a permanent character, such as a business or political community.

Such use of community art always includes strengthening resilience—that is, the ability to withstand even stressful situations—and promotes a sense of coherence (Schiffer, 2001, p.11). Community art is committed to a salutogenetic approach (Bengel *et al.*, 1998). Metaphorically, community art could be said to strengthen a community's immune system so that members or collectives of the community can respond early to conflicts before they escalate.

The instructions for decentering within such a situation can be borrowed from art-oriented events, as it requires creative work from a large number of people and at the same time can become an alternative experience of the world for the community. As possibilities, some forms may be pointed out:

- a mural or mosaic of fired tiles, with a vernissage
- a dance theater with your own music improvisation group for an anniversary
- a performance for the beginning of spring or similar seasonal celebrations, such as New Year or Easter, including all types of art
- a parade with motifs, costumes, and masks at carnival time
- a garden or park design with installations.

The difference between an event organized as a decentering and an entertainment event is the approach, which in the decentering always envisages a concern, dignifies the event with an aesthetic analysis, and includes a harvest.

Team consulting

Working with teams differs from working with groups in several ways. Common to both is that the counselor addresses not only the individuals present but also the team as a whole and possibly additionally individual sub-groups that result from the organizational structure or become apparent in the course of the first contacts. In addition, the overarching system that connects the individual team members—for example, the department or the institution as a whole—must always be kept in mind.

In contrast to the group coming together for a session for the first time, the counselor encounters a "well-rehearsed team" in the first team meeting—and he may encounter a myth at the same time. The team can be described as "well-rehearsed" because the individual members are connected more or less by a shared history. In the course of this history, unofficial hierarchies have emerged alongside official ones. Working communities, friendships, occasionally love affairs, but also more or less pronounced enmities have developed. There are alliances and coalitions. Only some of these structures and patterns are generally known, with some being talked about openly; others are never mentioned, even though all team members know about them.

"The team" as a well-functioning, close-knit working community is, however, unfortunately often largely a myth that exists primarily in the head of the team leader. It can be described as a myth because, for example, the team as a whole hardly ever sees each other, or individual team members rarely work together for individual, organizational, or task-related reasons.

There are advantages if the counselor is aware of the general specifics of a team before starting to work with it. On the other hand, in our experience, it only plays a minor role whether this work is called "team supervision," "team consulting," or "team development." What is decisive is the specification of the concrete assignment.

What is up for discussion when working with teams? It is the team-internal relationships, the personal and given scope of role design, certain team-internal regulations such as breaks, work distribution, and the like; in addition, certain work processes, sessions, functions, departments, possibly even mission statements, and goals or parts thereof. In principle, team-internal rules (open and hidden, e.g., "If you're not for it, you're against it"), formal and informal structures (e.g., how the "old" treat the "young" or how the founding figures are treated), and other aspects of the team culture are also available. The connection with the conditions in the overarching system parts that cannot be directly influenced in the work with the team must always be taken into account.

Teams seek the help of an outside expert for practical solutions to problems in fundamentally difficult situations (e.g., after restructuring or when many new employees have to be integrated) or to improve team spirit. Support is also often sought for better coping with recurring, difficult work situations and thus for further professionalization of the work performed.

Based on our fundamental approach to working with people and the resource-oriented orientation, some principles have proven to be especially useful in working with teams.

Care should be taken to ensure that everyone present has a chance to speak, so that entire phases of the conversation are not dominated by "speakers."

It is helpful to observe implicit rules of conversation or to introduce them explicitly.

At the beginning of the joint work, it is often helpful to take a relatively broad inventory. This should include the team's accomplishments, strengths, and shared joys. It seems to be useful that team strengths are brought up before an upcoming issue is discussed in detail.

The verbalized or otherwise visible appreciation by the supervisor or coach is also valuable in work with teams. This appreciation must be expressed first and foremost to the entire team, but also to the team leader who may be present and in a balanced form to individual team members.

Formulated and concretized goals and visions of goals give direction to the joint work and strengthen the motivation of those involved. In parallel, it is also important to record the goals already achieved and to collect together everything that has proved helpful with regard to their achievement.

In the solution- and resource-oriented approach, interpretations of problem behavior are gently interrupted, especially if they could lead to scapegoating. At best, they can be left as one possible hypothesis among many. The focus of the joint work is primarily on the steps towards a desired future and on what strengthens and supports such steps.

Humor and the allowing of humor also support the work with teams.

Artistic and playful means get team members out of their chairs and create "movement" for that reason alone. This can facilitate a change of perspective. Moreover, in a nonverbal form of presentation, additional aspects often become visible that were not encountered in the previous conversation.

In our work with teams, we use, among other things, forms of simple movement sequences or sounds and rhythms to tune in together at the beginning of a session. Sociometric constellations allow team members to get to know each other in a completely different way and make commonalities, differences, and groupings visible. Post-it notes on the wall, labeled with words or symbols, make the difference of viewpoints or the multitude of possible situations visible and can also be easily and vividly arranged, grouped, and regrouped during processing. Symbolic objects, such as symbols of team strengths, which are placed in the room at the beginning of the session, can be referred to metaphorically during the work.

The appreciation associated with this is much better accepted than verbal praise. An artistically designed installation work with mutual good wishes at the beginning of the year, joint artistic work at a festive occasion, or as an expression of a joint mourning process strengthen the cohesion and mutual bond and can contribute significantly to the reorganization and transformation of the team culture.

The method of Intermodal Decentering is not easy to apply to work with teams. Practitioners argue that there is usually not enough time for a carefully executed decentering in all parts, followed by an aesthetic analysis, a phase of harvesting, and transfer into the team's everyday life, because, in each phase, all participants have to be involved in the work. This is undoubtedly true when only two or two and a half hours are available for teams with eight or more people. We, therefore, tend to schedule only half-day or full-day sessions with medium or larger teams and see them less frequently in return. This is because, according to our observations, Intermodal Decentering can also have a very beneficial effect in teams.

Working on a collaborative artwork clearly and sustainably changes the atmosphere in a team. For example, within a sluggish, difficult discussion phase, the team members present are asked to do something together that they have never done before in this way, and thus often get to know completely new sides of themselves and others. The professional must, however, keep the level of challenge of the task in check. What is to be worked on within the decentering must not overtax anyone and must nevertheless allow for a satisfying and appealing work. The task must also not be too easy; otherwise, the participation will quickly become casual for some of the participants and lose all appeal.

For Intermodal Decentering with a team, it is imperative that the work succeeds. Even in decentering, a team remains itself—namely, a multi-person system that is judged in everyday life according to its performance and also judges itself accordingly.

Not infrequently, a successful work triggers obvious astonishment among those involved: "Fantastic, what we've achieved!" "We're not so bad!" Many are proud of what has been achieved in a very short time through joint effort. Thus, the novel shared experience alone creates a mood of success and confidence.

At the end of a session with decentering, the team members very often leave the room in a completely different mood; they laugh, seem exhilarated—and this even if, due to a lack of time, the transfer phase, which is particularly important for a team, could not be completed in all parts. The success at the end of a session is likely to be helped by the harvest, which is usually very rich in teams, and shows—even if not yet in detail—the variety of perspectives and thus the many fundamentally possible solutions.

Even if the concrete solution has not yet been worked out in detail, the relief in the team is often palpable. On one occasion, team members took care of the discussed problem on the staircase on their way out through bilateral, time-limited agreements, and then reported on it almost casually at the next meeting.

The use of decentering when working with teams requires special care. It can be assumed that one cannot decenter from the team structure as such. It remains even in the decentering phase.

Therefore, it is important to construct the task appropriately and formulate it specifically. Within the decentering, the task should exclusively use the terms of the corresponding artistic tradition. For example, the instructions always speak of the "ensemble" or the "performing arts company." It is recommended to propose mainly improvisations or designs that require an ensemble performance. Special attention must be paid to the distribution of tasks.

The distribution of the tasks—for example, in the theater, the tasks of stage management, script, costumes, light, and roles—should be given or directed in such a way that it does not cause the problem formulated in the concern. The various artistic media available are suited in different ways to set up the task in such a way that this danger can be avoided. For example, a musical improvisation in an ensemble will require a completely different performance from the participants than the construction of a forest hut. In the former, the elaboration happens through making music and requires unfamiliar arrangements during the musical process. The "Construction Company," on the other hand, needs a prior distribution of tasks, ranging from architecture to the procurement of materials. The situation is different again with dance improvisation or a mural.

In general, it can be said that such decisions have a more significant decentering effect, the more they occur in the course of the respective improvisation itself. Nevertheless, the preceding discourses or instructions for the distribution of tasks on stage or in the studio can serve exceptionally well as bridges from everyday life into the world of art.

If the chosen medium is particularly unfamiliar to some of those present, a stimulating introduction to the medium may be useful. We recommend the use of instructions and constructions that reflect the facilitator's preferences in the particular art area. It is then easier to let one's enthusiasm flow into the introduction.

If specific roles are represented in the team—for example, if the team leader is present—this should also be taken into account. It is certainly possible to choose an ensemble or company structure analogous to the structure of the team. However, this arrangement carries the risk that the problems formulated in the previous discussion will reappear in the decentering.

When it comes to particular roles in the team, it is very instructive for them to have new experiences and surprises during the alternative world experience and within the play in unfamiliar posts. This is also true when a structure similar to the team is planned, but then the typical people do not take over these particular roles.

However, it must always be ensured that all those present have their say. This applies to all parts of the joint work, especially to the processing of the decentering task, the aesthetic analysis, and the phase of harvesting. The vote of each person present is important, as long as they are committed to the task. Each person must explicitly state their willingness to "do something different" before the decentering phase and then be allowed to contribute something meaningful to the joint work, even if they are unable—for example, for physical reasons—to participate in all parts.

Special attention must be paid to the transfer of aspects from the harvesting phase into the team's everyday life. It takes time to formulate concrete, realizable conclusions from an association from the harvest phase that particularly appealed. In addition, it is usually not the case that the same association is in the foreground for all team members.

If there is not enough time in the session for this process, one possibility might be to require, as homework, a list of possible concrete conclusions from each person present for the next session. This formally postpones dealing with the problematic situation, but dealing already with "conclusions" is likely to change individual behavior in the corresponding situation.

If there is a lack of time, we tend to have better experiences if we do not process the results of the harvesting phase and their different weighting by individual team members at all, but instead strengthen the team's self-efficacy forces in the final phase of the session. This can be done, for example, by highlighting again in a special way the potentials of the team that have become visible in the artistic work.

In summary, it can be stated that decentering in work with teams not only has positive effects on finding solutions but also positively influences team spirit and team identity, thereby supporting the further development of a stimulating and mutually supportive team culture. However, the implementation of a decentering process needs sufficient time. This factor should not be underestimated. If sessions cannot be extended beyond two and a half hours, an additional option is to work with pre-announced decenterings occasionally. This means that a decentering is announced or agreed upon for the next session. On the day of the session itself, the introductory rounds and clarification of the issue can and should be kept as short as possible, so that, with the explicit agreement of all present, the decentering can begin, for example, after only half an hour.

7.2 Limits

In principle, limits arise when there are dangers involved for someone or something or when the procedure appears to be unfeasible or ineffective. This also applies to the work with Intermodal Decentering.

At this point, however, it must be emphasized that we have by no means had concrete experience with our method and decentering with all potential client groups at the time of writing this book. Thus, we cannot say anything about its application in childhood and early adolescence or in severe mental or intellectual impairment cases.

Psychological danger as a limit

In principle, the situation in Intermodal Decentering is the same as in all methods where work is done primarily through the connection between the professional and the client. This means that every therapeutic professional must have therapeutic training in order to be able to intervene appropriately in critical moments. This is especially true in the clinical field.

In contrast to most confrontational methods, at least some of the time, our conversational approach emphasizes the client's strengths and successes. However, at the same time, we also take the suffering and inadequacies seriously in an appreciative way. In artistic activity, we work according to the principle of "low-skill-high-sensitivity" to achieve a sense of achievement. Our experience shows that the vast majority of our clients feel not only understood but generally strengthened and supported by this methodical approach. It is not uncommon for us to observe physical reactions of joyful surprise during the sessions.

However, the professional must be aware that the effect of such an extremely positive reaction can quickly level off again outside the counseling room. It, therefore, seems necessary to point out a possible "cooling off" in an appropriate way or to give a corresponding homework assignment so that the disappointment is not experienced as doubly painful.

(SUPPOSEDLY) LIMITED APPLICATION POSSIBILITY

From professional colleagues who have only recently become familiar with the approach to work presented here, one hears again and again the statement: "Not feasible...with these people (in these situations) I can't ...after all." They think of leaving the usual counseling setting through artistic or playful activity and working with respecters, with clients much older than the counselor; or they think of working with clients with particular disabilities and limitations. Our experience so far does not confirm these fears. They are likely to be mostly internal barriers in the counselor herself. The counselor does not feel secure enough to work with certain clients using a method that is very unfamiliar to her professional background.

In any case, it makes sense to pay attention to such barriers and to take them seriously. At the same time, it must be remembered that it always takes courage to introduce something new and unfamiliar into the work. From a professional point of view, it can be stated that the described approach cannot be expected to have any real adverse effects, as long as there is an open, sensitive, and reasonably sustainable relationship basis between client and professional. There may indeed be situations in which a conversation with a complete decentering phase is not possible. Nevertheless, even there, elements of a resource-oriented approach and art and play can probably be used with good and lasting success.

UNSUITABLE SITUATIONS

Here, too, it should be emphasized that we have too little experience at this point to be able to make a comprehensive statement on this point.

There are, on the other hand, three different initial situations in which the use of decentering is not indicated or is indicated only in exceptional cases. First and foremost, there are the concerns of clients who primarily require professional advice—that is, where the focus is on the exchange of know-how and information. However, as soon as personal aspects of the person seeking advice come into play, a phase of decentering can even be beneficial in this situation.

In the very first session with a previously completely unknown client, we are very cautious about using decentering. This is especially true if working with artistic or playful means is unfamiliar in the professional field in question.

A whole other limit lies in the person of the counselor himself. Anyone who always wants to keep all the strings in his hand in counseling, who wants to know all the possible consequences before taking each next step, and who has trouble dealing with the unexpected and surprises, will have a hard time with the way of working described in this book. Such a limit must also be taken seriously—always in the knowledge that, in principle, it can be widened.

INEFFECTIVENESS OF THE METHOD AS A LIMIT

Although we have been working with this approach for more than ten years now, we can say comparatively little on this point. As already mentioned, our work—and that of former students from whom we receive feedback—focuses on adults, with the exception of those with severe mental or intellectual impairments. In this clientele, positive effects of decentering work are practically always observed, often even those that can be described as actual turning points in the process. To appreciate the horizon of experience so far, however, it must be pointed out that we by no means include a decentering phase in every session.

As a matter of principle, there must also be situations in which Intermodal Decentering is not effective. Miracle cures are notoriously untrustworthy. Therefore, below are some more situations where Intermodal Decentering has not been shown to be ineffective, but it has limited effectiveness, and its application, therefore, needs to be carefully considered. It is difficult when clients find it hard to get out of a habitual problem-laden pattern in order to engage with what is happening in a curious, discovering, and exploratory way. We then usually stay longer with the resource-oriented conversation and design the decentering phase in a straightforward, unpretentious way.

We also reach limits when the problem to be worked on implants itself in the decentering phase and becomes the focus of attention.

A situation of this kind once manifested itself in a training setting as follows.

> In the training group, the student who made herself available as a client describes in her concern how, when faced with challenges that she likes and enjoys (educational assignments, facilitation, etc.), she is always blocked and has nothing more to say.
>
> As a vision, she formulates, "Implementation is the topping of the preparatory work." A good outcome within the current session

would be if she can laugh at herself. Inadvertently, we do not talk about exceptions, and also strengths are not mentioned in the conversation part before the decentering phase.

Counselor and client agree on the art form of theater for decentering. The client wants to work on a comedy.

During the decentering, she suddenly says, when she wants to enter the stage again, that she is now exactly in the situation where "it" blocks. Thus, the problem has installed itself in the decentering phase. We try to change the direction and the role of the "scriptwriter." The result is that it gets worse. The client becomes a "theater case" (an actress with a performance block during the show).

It seems reasonable to assume that the concern was not sufficiently included in the preparation for this decentering—for example, no experiences of positive coping were brought up. Perhaps another artistic form of expression, less similar to the problem situation described, would have been more favorable. Finally, it must be considered that in this problem situation, any decentering that is designed as a demonstration within a training group is basically "theme-near" and requires special care, as explained in Chapter 4.

OTHER LIMITS AND CONSTRAINTS

Our kind of decentering makes demands on the practice space and its equipment. It goes without saying that someone who wants to create something with a client needs to have appropriate material available, and someone who wants to create with movement needs appropriate space.

It may also be difficult in the case of culturally based restrictions on artistic expression, such as the taboos on images in a specific religious environment. This must also be taken into account in the case of impaired affective ability, such as in the case of severely traumatized people or people who are in an acute phase of mourning. In such situations, we as process leaders are challenged to create something meaningful even with minimal expression (minimal art).

Decentering relies on the relaxed, curious, open attitude of the counselor. If she does not feel able to do this, it is more appropriate to work in a way in which she feels safe. On the other hand, our experience shows that most people in the Western world are willing to engage as clients, get involved, and then participate to an amazing degree.

It is also helpful to pick people up in their everyday life and their own world. Bringing the self-evident into new references and thereby making it innovative so that it can be reflected in everyday theories, avoiding any technical jargon, is almost always an effective approach. Example:

> A chair installation, which is tried out with the generally well-known instructions of the Rheumatism League for sitting down and standing up, prompts shaping of movement and can then lead to a chair scene with mimic dance theater. Interestingly, it turns out time and again that clients are already largely won over when everyday things are presented in a surprising, unfamiliar way.

8

The Origins

8.1 The phenomenological thinking and the development of the art-oriented practice

The work-oriented method in the field of art therapies

The work-oriented approach in art-oriented therapy and counseling is a further development of the interdisciplinary art therapies that were introduced in the early 1970s at Lesley University in Cambridge, Massachusetts. This approach understands the artistic process always as a towards-work, where each work has its own way of being completed or, as a child would say, "finished." Even if a work is not completed, it is still part of the essence of this artistic process that there is something that wants to be completed, something that "speaks to us" or "tells us something." Meanwhile, from these beginnings, different expressions have emerged in different fields of work. They are summarized in the English-language literature as "expressive arts" (EXA) in consulting, counseling, psychotherapy, supervision, and coaching and organized in associations. In German, we also find "expressive arts (EXA)," the term "*kunst- und expressiveorientierte Psychotherapie, Bildung, Beratung, und Therapie.*"[1]

This book is based on the method developed in the 1990s, which uses the structural relationship of the individual arts in the design

---

1 For example, in the International Expressive Arts Therapy Association (IEATA) and in a training network, the International Network of Expressive Arts Therapy Training Centers. Nationally, the corresponding groups are often integrated as a specialty in one of the associations for the art therapies or psychotherapy. In Switzerland, for example, in the "*Schweizer Fachverband für Gestaltende Psychotherapie und Kunsttherapie*" (GPK) and in the "*Schweizer Charta für Psychotherapie.*"

process with clients. This intermodal structural principle and the challenges it poses to the designer have been increasingly seen in relation to the challenges a problem poses to the client. An analogy can be drawn between the creative process of transforming the unformed and the task that the client has to solve. By focusing on the unformed in the artistic process, the client can be encouraged to shift away from their "deformed" problem, potentially leading to a positive outcome.

Centering/decentering was then first conceptualized by Margo Fuchs (1994)[2] from the structure of the intermodal group process.

The work-oriented method, on the other hand, has been developed out of "aesthetic responsibility" (Knill, 1995, 1999). We understand this as the responsibility of the therapist or counselor towards the work and its process of creation.

It is these approaches that have then been enriched and expanded to include the process of Intermodal Decentering. While work-oriented work is possible from various metatheoretical positions, decentering presupposes a certain conception of humanity and a corresponding metatheory. We use the abbreviation "art-oriented methods" for the basic approaches of the interdisciplinary method of artistic therapy and counseling.

The holistic view

It was not so long ago that headaches, for example, were attributed either causally to a chemical process or exclusively to a psychological imbalance. It was only after the middle of the last century that people increasingly considered possible connections between physical and psychological disorders, and even genetic, environmental, social, and family-related factors were increasingly taken into account as influences. The cause–effect principle, which directly attributed each effect to a cause, now gave way to a notion of interdependent effect factors that triggered different consequences depending on the conditions. This so-called holistic, integrative approach was a major impetus for the formation of an interdisciplinary direction in art therapies.

---

2 "De-Centering": Experimental learning, the intermodal laboratory, forming, unforming de-forming through artistic mediums and expression (Fuchs, 1994).

While the body therapy approach had a strong influence on the development of the integrative approach of "expressive arts" (EXA) for reasons to be elaborated, the inclusion of the social environment and systems theory thought initially played only a minor role.

The art therapies already organized at that time included music therapy, creative therapy, dance and movement therapy, drama therapy, psychodrama, and poetry therapy. They were mainly based on the well-known psychotherapeutic schools. For example, there was psychoanalytic dance therapy, Jungian art therapy, humanistic creativity therapy, and behavioral music therapy. With the assumption that, in the holistic approach, every action also presupposes the body, physical expression gained importance. The artistic action also presupposes the physical.

Artistic expression in the creative action is hardly conceivable without the use of physical movement and highly sensitive being-with-the-senses. In its perception and expression, artistic activity is always concerned with physical things, whereby this physical aspect comes to the fore in a differentiated way depending on the art discipline. Here, a broad spectrum of indicative considerations offered itself for the advisory and therapeutic approach. Which treatment circumstances indicate consideration of using the body in dance as a design object, and when is the more haptically and optically oriented modeling with clay appropriate, which distances itself physically from the one creating it?

In the body-oriented therapies at that time, among other things, access to the not-lived was sought through bodily expression. As an intervention, exercise-like procedures and settings were preferred that activated breath, voice, and movement and evoked direct bodily expressions (laughing, crying, screaming, trembling, etc.). These were in turn explored in the conversation for insights and then integrated. Many of these made reference to Wilhelm Reich and, theoretically, to the early publications of Breuer and Freud. Catharsis was at the center. For example, Lowen's bioenergetics developed a unique body analysis, and Janov's primal therapy proposed an analysis and regression theory focused on the client's early childhood phase and employed dramatic re-experiencing as a method.

An exception was the psychodrama of Moreno, which developed its own theory and cultivated in the theater a culturally anchored form of expression oriented to the actual life situation in order to then also enable a catharsis-oriented integration.

In the development of the art- and expressiveness-oriented methods, psychodrama had a kind of bridging function (at Lesley University, for example, with Peter Rowen and Zerka Moreno). In Norway and Israel, psychodrama centers integrated the EXA approach, and some EXA trainers are still well-known psychodramatists today.

From the beginning, fundamental considerations led the art- and expressiveness-oriented method to understand the client's expression as a body–soul phenomenon in an anthropological context. Thus, it distinguished itself from the purely body-oriented therapies in the following ways.

Artistic expression belongs to the human being as an existential. It is not a symptom of a disorder, but a natural, holistic mode of expression. Purposeful exercises to achieve specific sense-expressed effects were discarded as mechanistic. In the process, however, catharsis—that is, "purification" through an adequate "removal" of what makes one ill—was initially welcomed, something similar to psychodrama. In contrast to the exclusively body-oriented therapies, a form of expression that is inherent to the nature of art began to emerge on its own. There has to be more breathing when singing a text than when speaking it; a dance of joy can be experienced energetically and bodily/emotionally better than the sentence "I feel joy."

Since artistic expression was seen as a human existential and not symptomatic of pathological development, the basis also included attention to health and the importance of resources. Very early on, the resulting works were seen as assisting or helpful spirits that could be accessed by the client beyond the sessions and used as a form of mental exercise, such as being looked at, recited, sung, whistled, or practiced.

Artistic expression is to be understood as something that is physical and sensorial but always also imaginative. The symbolic content of artistic expression is therefore just as crucial as the body-sense experience of expression. This makes it culturally anchored and comprehensible to others, especially to observers, therapists, and group members. The content is related to cultural heritage, to our stories, pictures, songs, music, films, and poetry. The reductionist reinterpretation of symbolic content by psychological or spiritual metatheories was vehemently rejected early on (Knill, 1986). The "responding conversation" to and with the artistic work was paramount, and, in early publications, was referred to as a "dialogue with the arriving" image (McNiff, 1988). A major role was played by Blake, who, as a poet, thinker, and painter, castigated the "one-dimensionality" of "the singular explanatory myths" and, so to speak, historically anticipated postmodernism with the thesis of "multiple narratives" (cf. Callahan, 1992).

The fact that artistic creation is a disciplined play in cultural traditions (music or theater, mourning and pleasure play, etc.) led to the study of theories of play and to the proximity to play therapy for children.

The basic considerations, which in the art and expressiveness-oriented method placed the body–soul view in an anthropological context, led to an interdisciplinary approach for various reasons.

Artistic expression belongs to humanity like language. However, it is a language of a different kind. Poetry, in its innovative use of words, can thus be seen as "thinking of a different kind" (Fuchs, 2002, p.162). In all spontaneous artistic activities, not only are all senses continuously engaged but various modes of reflection are also required. This always happens in the context of what is just revealed in the act of shaping. In the process, if it is musically realized, a text may appear in a different cultural context in connection with the melody. A dance "says" additional things through the rhythm of the music chosen for it. The sensitive being-with-the-senses in artistic activity, or in artistic "language," manifests itself differently in the various art disciplines. The use of the voice and the body in music is fundamentally different from writing and reading a text, forming a sculpture, or playing on stage, and yet they are all part of a body–soul expression.

These considerations called for an *interdisciplinary understanding* in counseling and therapy. An interdisciplinary attitude is intrinsically part of the artistic tradition. Thus, even though it is usually considered a discipline in its own right, dance is not conceivable without an understanding of music or the scenic, just as poetry, while belonging to the realm of language, cannot be thought of without rhythm and images.

The interdisciplinary considerations also referred to the idea of the *Gesamtkunstwerk* (total work of art), whose philosophical foundations

Richard Wagner related to Feuerbach and Schopenhauer. Wagner understood the *Gesamtkunstwerk* as a total expression of art under the guidance of poetry. He composed the music, wrote the text, designed the stage set, even the opera house, choreographed the work, and then conducted it himself (Szeemann, 1983).

What happens when a text comes to an image or a mask finds language? Under what circumstances or conditions should a particular art discipline be chosen and in what form? Not only do these questions affect all art disciplines, but they also have cultural, anthropological, physiological, and psychological aspects, as well as epistemological considerations.

The anthropological view was also devoted to the folk ritual as well as linguistic formulations. In the German-language area, the phrase "*künstlerische Ader*" (artistic vein) brought attention to one's creative, capabilities that are separate from any academic artistic talents. Also, in all these ideas, just as in popular festivities, the boundary between the artistic disciplines and general creative activity is blurred. For example, the decoration of the stage at the village jubilee and the music for the gymnastic round dance on this stage are created entirely by amateurs, so to speak "interdisciplinarily," in collaboration. One of the everyday experiences of the blurring of boundaries between the classical art disciplines and their interdisciplinary networks is the intermedial linking of image, text, music, and movement in today's predominant visual media of video and film. Intermodal art and expressive therapy have therefore been intensively engaged with these interdisciplinary media from the very beginning, studying them in context and using them productively.

As a result, the interdisciplinary approach to art therapies followed the maxim that we must start from the client's point of view when choosing the means of creation. This requires from the therapist, in addition to the therapeutic qualifications, a certain breadth of artistic skills in order to be able to meet clients in a motivating way. It has been shown that performance art can be an excellent training ground for acquiring this breadth.

From the very beginning, performance artists are familiar with the interdisciplinary nature of their art. Their art usually has a focus. Often the artists come from the visual arts, but also from music, film, theater, dance, and increasingly poetry. In their quest for personal expression, they do not limit themselves to mere techniques; performance artists always want to take into account the current state of the arts and the diversity of all artistic possibilities. The quality of a performance is, therefore, a balancing act between interdisciplinary virtuosity and authentic expression. The play between music, performing arts, dance, theater, body expression, and back again is subject to a constant process of evaluation. Mastering this play requires the artist to be extraordinarily empathetic and constantly present while keeping an eye on the interactions between the various art disciplines and materials.

The exploratory search for the most effective material is not limited to a single art discipline. When a material, such as a theatrical prop or a piece of clothing, is found in one art discipline, it is subjected to a thorough examination by elements of another discipline—for example, the process of danced movement to various musical sketches—until it fits the form, content, and expression of the whole performance.

Understandably, a therapeutic setting oriented in this way along the lines of performance art was soon seen as very complex, since it was a matter not only of shaping the relationship between therapist and client but also of enabling a creative process that was always intended to express something work-like, which in turn entered into a connection with all those involved. This work-like quality was considered essential from the beginning since what is designed is present as an object— a designed "something" that can be seen and heard in its reality by all participants, a manifestation that can be experienced by the senses, and which also always refers to other works. A lament is culturally anchored in the laments of the client's culture. Images always have references to other images. This is true for all designed objects. In this way, there is always a twofold reference—a reference to one's own experience and a reference to the world, and thus also a kind of distancing from the purely self-referential.

For readers interested in the history of science, the main impulses that led to a theoretically founded method are mentioned here in keywords.

The intermodal method received essential impulses in connection with the turn to the phenomenon of imagination in artistic expression from James Hillmann, the founder of archetypal psychology, who participated in the formation of theory as a visiting professor at Lesley University (Knill, 1995). The *crystallization principle* (see the explanations in the next section "The theories and principles of the intermodal method"), which builds on the imagination modalities of image, movement, word, action, and sound/rhythm, emerged from this collaboration.

The developmental psychological considerations of Piaget, introduced by Knill, had a strong influence on the formation of theory, offering a theoretical bridge between the various disciplines of artistic activity as well as the body, movement, and thinking. The art-oriented methods for guiding and accompanying artistic processes are based on the realization that movement intelligence forms the basis for all more complex thinking and that discovering experimentation in motivating play spaces can bring surprising insights. One result of these considerations can be found in the theory of the "low-skill–high-sensitivity" method of instruction, which makes it possible to work in artistic ways with people who have no prior artistic experience.

From the beginning, music educators and therapists had a significant influence, which may be explained by the understanding of music as a *Gesamtkunstwerk*. Among the leading theorists of this direction are Hans-Helmut Decker-Voigt (1983), Paolo Knill (1979), and Wolfgang Roscher (1980). With his Lesley Institute for Media and Expressive Therapy in Hösseringen (Lower Saxony), Decker-Voigt developed fundamental principles of an intermedial professional training and later implemented them at the University of Music and Theater in Hamburg.

Of particular interest was *polyaesthetics* as represented by Wolfgang Roscher (Mozarteum Salzburg) (Schwarzbauer, 2001). This is the approach of a multimedia art practice, which first proved itself in integral music education. It reflects the interdisciplinary, intercultural, historical, and social practice and perception of art. The approach has been extended in the therapeutic direction (Mastnak, 1993). Polyaesthetics has been particularly instrumental in differentiating sensorial expression and perception, taking into account the multimedia practice of art, and has shed light on archaic aspects in the practice of various artistic media. It has had a significant influence on intermodal theory.

The theory and practice of the interdisciplinary approach initially also borrowed heavily from body-oriented therapy practiced in the studio or atelier. From theater and dance, it was Alec Rubin (therapist and director in New York, "Theater of the Encounter") who served as an adjunct professor at Lesley University and taught an intermedial and strongly body-oriented drama and dance therapy modeled on the theater laboratory of Jerzy Grotowski. Studio, atelier, and stage were central to the transformative experience for Shaun McNiff (from the visual arts) and Paolo Knill (from music and performance art). They were also not to be compromised in the therapeutic setting. A "Theory Indigenous to Art" was postulated (Knill, 1986). McNiff formulated art-based theory and research with Fuchs in the Lesley University Thesis Seminar, which later led to the concept of "Art-Based Research" (McNiff, 1998).

In this context, the influence of Rudolf Arnheim is also important (Levine, 2002, pp.266–282) with his perceptual aesthetics developed from Gestalt psychology (Köhler, Koffka, Wertheimer). Arnheim was invited to Lesley University on various occasions and participated in the theoretical discourse of the faculty. His opinion of art therapies was very positive but pointed: art is directed to the world and not to the self; artistic activity is first of all devoted to a shaping to be universally witnessed by others and not so much to self-expression. Arnheim values the senses highly; the work reveals itself aesthetically through the senses. Meaning or sense-making emerges through the interplay of structure and form in the work. This discourse was instrumental in the formulation of theory around "Aesthetic Commitment" and "Aesthetic Resonance" (Knill, 1995)—that is, foundations necessary for the work-related method.

The founding faculty of Lesley University also turned to the *phenomenological model of thought* of Binswanger and Boss in an effort to interpret art in a way that was appropriate to the art the founding faculty of Lesley University furthermore turned to the phenomenological model of thought of Binswanger and Boss. Medard Boss (1982) was an honorary member of the Artist Therapist Association (later dissolved into an international association). In the 1980s, the focus of phenomenological research and theory building shifted to Europe, predominantly Switzerland. In the process, a differentiated, independent school of psychotherapy developed (art- and expressiveness-oriented psychotherapy—ISIS), which distinguished itself within the "Swiss Charter for Psychotherapy" with its phenomenological orientation. At the same time, a counseling model has also emerged ("Supervision as Art"—EGIS). With regard to the art-oriented orientation, the latter was committed to work-related practice from the beginning and developed in connection with the solution-oriented turn towards Intermodal Decentering (IDEC®).

The theories and principles of the intermodal method

The crystallization principle (Knill, 1990b/2002) refers to the core of the individual arts and states that the arts are intermodal, but in each case with specific characteristics. In each art medium, a certain aspect comes to the fore: thus, in music, sound and rhythm crystallize first and foremost; that is, music cannot be thought of without sound and rhythm, even though it can move, incorporate texts, and evoke inner images.

In all art disciplines, we find a number of sensory and communicative modalities. In the visual arts, for example, we know that the sensorimotor and tactile senses are involved. We know that a painting does not communicate through visuals alone but also through the rhythms of color. A painting may also evoke a story or describe an action.

Music, on the other hand, as already pointed out, involves not only the auditory senses but also the sensorimotor, kinetic, tactile, and visual senses. Music communicates through rhythm and sound, through words and rhymes that can evoke inner images.

Despite the interdisciplinary nature of all the arts, it is instructive to distinguish the various art disciplines according to the predominant modalities they each seem to favor. The crystallization principle also helps in differentiating modalities of imagination. Each individual art discipline has its own vessels for clarification and sense-making, using the creative act as a vehicle for imagination within its own tradition in a specific, unique way. For example:

- It is possible to speak, dream, or talk without *images*, but images crystallize most clearly in a painting or sculpture. There is no visual art without images.
- One can be moved by music, as well as by a story or a

theatrical scene, or one can describe an action with a movement, but *movement* is best experienced through its crystallization in dance. There is no dance without movement.

- One may tell about *actions*, write about them, sing about them, or paint them, but the most impressive format to demonstrate an action is a scene on stage in the theater. There is no theater without action.
- One can walk rhythmically, move or speak, or one can communicate with sounds, by whistling or by grunting, but we experience sound and rhythm most intensely when they crystallize in *music*. There is no music without sound and rhythm.
- Words can be used to communicate visual images or to describe a scene or dramatic moments, but words best accentuate the poetic component of communication in *storytelling* or in a *poem*. There is no poetry without words.

The intermodal theory

This theory, developed in the context of the intermodal method in artistic expression, formulates the influence of the individual art disciplines and their specific practice on various aspects of a counseling or therapeutic connection. It distinguishes between interpersonal, intrapersonal, and transpersonal viewpoints (Knill, 1990b, pp.90–95).

Interpersonal aspects

The artistic disciplines regulate communication among the members of a group. We find restrictions through structure and form and facilitations of certain interactions that would be difficult outside the artistic form. Therefore, the process of a group can be made visible or audible and developed and encouraged through staging or choreography.

Moreno (1967) appreciated some of this in the psychodramatic practice of sociometry. If we compare the different disciplines of artistic expression in our intermodal practice, the differences can be elaborated. Painting and sculpting in groups facilitate the process of individuation because of their intrinsic move towards private, isolated creation. (An exception to this rule, however, would be the creation of a group painting or installation in which everyone can participate.)

Music, with its resounding, resonant presence that no one can avoid, tends to lead towards socialization. Dance and movement, on the other hand, open up possibilities for exploring the connections and coalitions within the group. When using different disciplines, the *intermodal transfer* can be well observed. Used correctly, it deepens or broadens expression, intensifies identification with the group, or, on the contrary, intensifies individuation. We thus offer possibilities that make people less afraid to find words that are beyond the ordinary, everyday conversation.

Intermedial transfer (*also change of media*)

Intermedial transfer refers to the change from one creative-artistic medium to another or the enrichment by additional artistic forms of expression (music to a poem) within the same medium.

The choice depends, apart from the resources of the involved person/s, on what presents itself through a holistic, sensory observation, what wants to be intensified, what is also still there, and what needs to be or should be clarified. Is it what moves, what resonates, what has formed an image, or what speaks in words?

Intrapersonal aspects

The most important intrapersonal aspects refer to the acquired emotional attitude of an individual or a collective towards a particular discipline of artistic expression. For example, some people have strong resistance to spontaneous expression through music, perhaps due to (remembered) stage fright from previous music lessons. Some cultures do not encourage spontaneous action because it might disrupt social order. Some of us are more comfortable with some forms of artistic expression than others, and these preferences may change with circumstances.

To illustrate, here are a few personal observations:

- When I examine myself and my habits, I see that I am used to painting a picture when I want to communicate an idea with clarity and accuracy.
- When I want to demonstrate a scene without long-winded comments and explanations, I use the magic of the theater. Maybe I play my grandmother, embodying her with my voice

and with characteristic gestures, imitating her sound when she called to the chickens: a kind of raven's cry that woke everyone on the farm in the morning.

- When I express myself through poetry, I feel most vulnerable. I write my most intimate notes or letters in poetic form.

Transpersonal aspects

Transpersonal aspects derive from the religious and ritual applications of the arts. Paintings, sculptures, and symbolic objects denote the place of worship and are like gateways to the place of sacred entities, the gods. Rather than casually discarding a painting of a client, it can be taken as a totem-like object for continued dialogue. For example, a painting may be hung like an altarpiece, or a sculpture of a client may "want" to be placed at the entrance to her home, giving the impression of protection there, or reminding her each time she comes home that she can leave some of the day's troubles outside.

Prayers are traditionally lyrical texts, and they lose none of their power through repetition. In fact, it is precisely repetition that is the essence of this experience so that they are memorized (known by heart). Such power lies in every touching poem. Who has not taken the time to read a love poem over and over again, renewing an emotional experience with each successive reading? It is, therefore, good practice in change processes to encourage repetition of what has been written (e.g., to suggest as homework the daily reading of a poem or story that came up in the session).

Dance and music are united in many ritual acts. Usually, the dance forms a bridge to theater-like productions, often with costumes or masks, while the music forms a link to the content of hymns and myths. The repeated staging of an important event (e.g., initiation, blessing, bonding, empowerment, transformation, birth, and death) occurs in dance and theatrical artistic vessels. It may be useful, therefore, to recall some of what has been achieved—for example, by revisiting or continuing a piece of music, song, dance, or scene—in a later session. Sometimes such a work is used each time as a conclusion, as a farewell, almost as a blessing, or at the beginning as a welcome.

As an inner voice, music can accompany us like a "positive ear-worm," rising helpfully in specific situations; sometimes, one begins to hum, whistle, or sing what was there as a work in a process of change. Surprisingly, such singing often changes the mood. Using art to effect change should not ignore the cultural traditions and creative practices from which it draws its power. To do so would be to dismiss one of the core sources of its strength in finding a solution.

8.2 The art- and expressiveness-oriented practice and the critique of other methods contained therein

The interdisciplinary theoretical orientation and the intermodal approach described above are fundamentally committed to a multidimensional understanding of meaning. That is, based on our constructivist thinking, we assign different meanings to a phenomenon. This practice, therefore, contradicts a reductive metatheoretical definition or interpretation of expression, as we find in many psychodynamically-oriented art therapies. Signs, symbols, and metaphors refer to themselves and not to "deeper things." The essence emerges from the thing itself coming to speech. Enrichment occurs through the avoidance of explanatory interpretations and the intensification of the responding attitude. The result of the expression is appreciated and explored in the here and now, in its richness, on the sensorial surface. Thus, the critique of art- and expressiveness-oriented practice also turns against mechanistic interpretive tendencies in art therapies of the New Age movement, which provide clients with symbolic meanings from, more or less ethnologically substantiated, categories of interpretation.

In the holistic approach of art- and expressiveness-oriented practice, we find on the one hand a critique of procedures that lose themselves in a singular approach (only deficit-oriented, only behavior-oriented, only trauma-oriented, etc.). On the other hand, there is a criticism of the holistic understanding of the New Age movement. As a concept, wholeness must remain intangible and imperfect since we in our imperfection are always included in the assumed wholeness. The intermodal approach is not a postulate for the integration of all arts with their existential manifestations. Through its interdisciplinary and intermodal orientation, it emphasizes sensitivity for both the commonalities and the differences, even if this leads to contradictions.

To the same extent, criticism is directed against an undue eclecticism in art therapies, which overlooks differences and contradictions out of a superficial tendency towards integration. In this kind of eclecticism, for example, it happens that different metatheories are interpreted in a fresh and cheerful manner. For example, in a picture, one speaks of "the energy" that is in this red, an energy that cannot unfold because this brown and black, on the upper left, somehow keep it in check, whereby it is also added that it looks as if the id is suppressed by strong superego forces.

Within expressive arts, however, the conversation is supposed to be about color and structure. So we could talk about this red as an expanding band, starting from the top in saturated purple and lightening into crimson, as it pours down; how the sharp edges, formed by the red and the almost black background, are softened by the sepia-brown, ornamental tendrils that look like stylized grapevines after cutting; and about what else surprisingly reveals itself in the work and became visible in the process.

The physical and sensorial approach taken by art- and expressiveness-oriented practice criticizes approaches that are exclusively cognitive, such as rational-emotive therapy (Ellis and Grieger, 1979). However, it places particular emphasis on the cognitive learning experience within the artistic accomplishment of the task set. This is a directly experiential, sensory one, which is usually evident in the client's mood and the tonus of his or her body. The art-oriented play range expansion allows structures of meaning, action, and thought to emerge that can be utilized. We also learn that clients can gain something like hope from the artistic process—a hopefulness that comes from the experience that in the process of moving towards the work, something always pulls towards completion. This can be understood teleologically as finding meaning in the beauty of the finished work (Knill, 2004, pp.269–284).

Artistic creation is assumed to be an existential. Thus, a resource orientation is initiated because existentials are implicitly assigned to the healthy. The art- and expressiveness-oriented method, therefore, criticizes a practice that is one-sidedly oriented towards pathology. In its development, the art-oriented method has also found application in dealing with pathology, although early publications spoke of the "contagiousness" of health in artistic activity (McNiff, 1988, pp.31–40; 1981, pp.29–45). In the step towards solution orientation (see Chapter 2), this resource-oriented aspect was then emphasized.

The pictorial or scenic representation of pain, for example, not only appears painful and sorrowful but also touches us through the beauty of the work (Picasso's *Guernica*, Käthe Kollwitz, the Passion plays and oratorios). Historically, this insight, which led to the formulation of "nurturing" beauty, was a step towards resource orientation. Later, the turn towards solution orientation happened.

Classical psychoanalytical art therapy has interpreted art as well as all other imaginative phenomena exclusively from the symbolic content, against the background of a narration related to pathology. The work-related direction of artistic therapies takes the artistic production as a creative achievement, independent of the content, and appreciates this fact.

Art- and expressiveness-oriented practice views artistic action as disciplined play in cultural traditions. This approach thus opens up to cultural anthropological considerations. The cycles of life and ways of being that are culturally anchored usually take on ritual artistic forms, such as baptisms, marriages, and celebrations of the dead. Cultural openness is inherent in art therapy in this way. Being aware of these traditions enables the individual to see himself in the context of the shared experience. The client is thus not exclusively at the mercy of his self-expression. He encounters the other and thus distances himself from the one-sided ego view within the cultural framework. This results in a critique of approaches that are detached from the cultural context or insensitively use ritual patterns from cultures foreign to the client, such as the use of a Japanese spirit ritual from the Shinto tradition to banish "negative energies" in a team development assignment of an organization committed to a European Christian tradition.

In the art- and expressiveness-oriented practice, the client is the starting point for the choice of creative means. We take into account that the client has more access to certain means than to others, and we take this fact seriously. We trust the client to find access to a design with his own resources, thus emphasizing his expertise. For example, a client who has only had negative experiences with music at school is given access to it by making installations or sculptures that can also create sound.

From this attitude, however, the art- and expressiveness-oriented practice also takes a critical position towards methods that are based on the deficits of the clients.

Introducing a third element into the existing dialogue between two parties can significantly alter the situation in a fundamentally new way, providing an expanded scope of action. The dialogue between the two is disrupted by its presence, allowing for new possibilities to arise. In this way, forms are critically questioned that are based exclusively on the intimacy of the encounter between two people in therapy. The emerging work is ultimately not controllable in detail in its emergence; that is, we engage in a process where the surprising not only becomes possible but is also desired. Such an attitude, in turn, contradicts all therapeutic approaches that tend towards a feasible (producible) therapeutic success, as is often the case in cognitive or purely behavioral approaches.

8.3 The Focus on Solutions practice and its tradition of thought

Focus on Solutions counseling is a distinctive step towards the client's autonomy. He is seen as an expert in his own life. If such a statement is not only declared but also practiced, this has implications for the counselor's position. However, before we turn to this topic and thus to the practice of solution orientation, we will take a brief historical flashback to the beginnings of psychoanalysis and its understanding of the doctor–patient connection, which was fundamentally new for the time.

Lorenzer (1984) describes the situation in Viennese psychiatry when Breuer and Freud went public with sensational case reports and theses. It is Vienna at the end of the 19th century, a time that was characterized, among other things, by a strong hierarchization. In contrast to earlier centuries, those suffering from so-called "nervous illnesses" are now almost universally regarded as sick. All authority thus rests with the physician, who, although he still knows very little about the clinical conditions with which he is confronted, nevertheless surrounds himself with an aura of scientificity. He is the person who speaks, perhaps asking some questions and then giving instructions. The patient speaks only when asked; otherwise, he is silent.

Freud's "analytic speech cure," which later developed into psychoanalysis, brings a striking turn in this respect. Here it is primarily the patient who speaks. The analyst sits behind him, listens, and remains silent for the most part. Lorenzer suspects that the reversal of these power relations contributed much more to the ostracism of Freud and his method in Viennese psychiatry than the assertion of the existence of early childhood sexuality.

Critically, from today's point of view, the "reversal of power relations" would probably only be described as a superficial one. The analyst of this generation is silent, but he knows that he knows better than his patient.

This is no longer the case in solution-oriented therapy. It thus goes a few steps further than Freud did back then. The solution-oriented approach to counseling views the client in a certain sense as an expert within the situation. By making this expertise visible, it supports it to solve the problems and difficulties at hand.

The behavioral approach according to Steve de Shazer

INITIAL STAGES

In the mid-1970s, a small team of family therapists led by Steve de Shazer in Milwaukee began to focus their commitment and innovative spirit on effective therapeutic interventions. The approach was pragmatic. The group accepted applications for therapy from patients from different cultures (individuals, couples, families) with clinical, social, educational, or addiction problems. One team member worked with each client while others sat behind the one-way mirror.

Many sessions were video-recorded. After establishing contact and an initial discussion phase, the session was always interrupted. During the break, the professionals involved exchanged their impressions and worked out the most effective intervention possible. The team member functioning as a therapist carried out the intervention and ended the session.

The next time, the effect of the intervention was reviewed. If an intervention showed useful results, it was used with other clients. If this revealed something like a pattern of an effective type of intervention, the team tried to explain it theoretically. This resulted in theoretical statements and, over time, a body of theory that slowly moved away from the other models prevalent at the time and was subsequently refined and further developed.

RESEARCH ON PRACTICE

From this approach, the logical conclusion was that time had to be reserved for specific practice research. Beginning in 1982, this research focused on observations that tasks prescribed to clients proved to be very helpful and useful in certain circumstances, even when they did not relate at all to the reported problem (e.g., Gingerich and de Shazer, 1991). In another research project, it was found that more than one-third of all enrollees experienced spontaneous improvements in their problem between the time of enrollment (usually by telephone) and the first session. The result was astonishing. In first meetings, the results could be included in interventions that were based precisely on these spontaneous improvements.

SYSTEMS THEORY BASIS

The members of the Milwaukee team came from systemically-oriented work with families. In the beginning, they were strongly influenced by the working methods of the Mental Research Institute (MRI) in Palo Alto, California, and its exponents Bateson (e.g., 1981), Satir (e.g., 1975), Watzlawick (e.g., Watzlawick *et al.*, 1969), and others. In an interview, Insoo Kim Berg, de Shazer's partner, reports that the original intention was to establish a second Palo Alto Institute in the Midwestern United States. This idea soon fell apart, as the team's meticulous observations showed that the prevailing theories of MRI at the time were far from confirmed in all cases. This largely unprejudiced observation practice in the team was fostered by the fact that the members came from very different backgrounds in their original professions. Insoo Kim Berg was originally a pharmacist, Steve de Shazer a musician and painter. The other early team members came from backgrounds in linguistics, sociology, and education. All had later undergone basic therapeutic training, many with a psychoanalytic background. They were all very impressed by the working methods and therapeutic successes of Milton Erickson (e.g., Rosen, 1985).

The resource- and solution-oriented approaches described in this book are also embedded in a basic systemic understanding. Section 6.3 provides insight into the related contexts.

When the experiences and observations were first published, they quickly caused a stir in the professional world (e.g., de Shazer, 1982). However, the detailed description of the procedure soon generated misunderstandings. The partly repetitive interventions, together with the high success rate, were understood as recipes, and the approach was subsequently qualified in part as rigid or even mechanistic. In the aforementioned interview, Insoo Kim Berg distances herself from such an understanding. The descriptions of the procedure may appear simple to the reader, but the procedure itself is by no means so. The therapeutic or counseling conversation is such a complex activity that it can never be reduced to isolated steps.

In order to give readers who are not familiar with the Focus on Solutions approach to consulting insight into this way of working, some basic assumptions and attitudes are presented below. This is not intended to be a complete description or even an appreciation of the work of the Milwaukee team. We will pick out what seems central to us, what has proven itself in our practical work, and what has been essential to the development of Intermodal Decentering. Those interested in the classical solution-focused counseling method are referred to the numerous professional literature (e.g., de Jong and Berg, 1998; Bamberger, 1999).

Assumptions, underlying attitude, and a misunderstanding

Central is everything that works

The Focus on Solutions approach is characterized by an almost uncompromising focus on what works and—in the opposite direction—a varying degree of moving away from everything that is problematic and difficult. Linguistically, the founders of this approach point out that the use of the word "problem" always implies the possibility of a solution or the existence of a "problem-free zone."

The importance of this kind of focalization of attention cannot be overestimated. It goes against both the habits of everyday life and what has characterized the Western counseling tradition so far.

In everyday life and in professional work, we are sensitive to difficulties and problems with which we are confronted. This applies to our dealings with ourselves and the people in our immediate environment as well as to professional practice. People who present themselves to us with problems deserve our attention. Both Western culture and professional tradition dictate that, as helpers, we approach suffering respectfully, get to know it, and explore it in all its interconnectedness, its depth, its origins, and its effects. This leads so far that some people define themselves largely or almost exclusively by their suffering, and, in a certain way, also distinguish themselves through it. It is not their perhaps modest abilities and talents that are important to them, not what they are still capable of achieving despite problems and difficulties, and certainly not the joys they experience that give them significance, but their problems with their multiple effects, their suffering, and pain.

It seems plausible that in our Western world, Christianity has played its part in this cultivation of suffering. It is also plausible that people generally deal with their suffering, difficulties, problems, and disorders more intensively than with their strengths and abilities or with what often, in an almost self-evident way and sometimes completely unnoticed, succeeds in their lives.

This culturally determined and, in many ways, seemingly natural tendency has been supported by traditional scientific thinking within counseling and therapy. Building on Western structuralist thinking, which sees what is encountered and visible or audible as merely an often-deceptive surface and assumes "the actual" and "the true" to be beneath the surface, "in the depths," a condition must be deeply grasped and understood if it is to be treated. It is necessary to get to the "core," to the "cause" of what is called a "symptom" (sign, characteristic, harbinger), if one wants to intervene effectively.

All this has left an impact on our clients and on us. It is a fact of experience that most of us can talk about our difficulties and problems in much greater detail and sophistication than we can about strengths, abilities, and what works. From this, I think we can conclude that most people in our culture are quite ignorant about the resources they have available to them. This is almost universally evident in daily counseling practice. Not only psychologically uninterested but even psychologically sensitized people are little aware of their strengths and know little about the underlying reasons for what works in their lives as if by itself.

If a work approach comes along that focuses almost exclusively on resources and strengths and is primarily interested in what succeeds, this triggers surprise and can be understood as an affront: "Is the seriousness of my situation being overlooked here?" a client might think. "Is the complexity of the problem situation being negated in a superficial way?" professionals might suspect. From our point of view, it should be emphasized that great attention must be paid to the cultivation of relationships in solution-focused practice and that the Focus on Solutions approach is not simply a methodical procedure among others, but for the professional is tied to a very fundamental change in the therapeutic attitude and way of working.

Consequently, the orientation of professional action towards resources and solutions has a major impact on the counselor's understanding of her profession in various fields of work. The professional working in therapy, for example, becomes a new expert in the activation of resources and the facilitation of healing processes. To be sure, she remains a professional therapist or supervisor, but the claim to be an expert in disorders and pathology is dropped. This is especially unfamiliar to professionals working in the field of medicine and also difficult for many social workers who, for example, are used to taking responsibility and solving problems for their clients in multi-problem situations. All professional counselors are now facing the new task of becoming "experts of a different kind" who can empower people to find their own solutions.

The client is the expert of his or her life

This is a logical consequence of the above. If I, as a professional, focus on what works, what I am looking for is to be found in the client and his environment. The resources are to be discovered there. They are not to be found in the professional, in their knowledge, or in reference books.

In this way, the client becomes an expert, even if he personally knows nothing about it and certainly does not know how to use his expertise. He is an expert on what is important and meaningful to him. He knows, or he has to find out what makes sense to him. He has experienced what works for him, what works and what doesn't, even if he does not remember it or did not pay much attention to it. This kind of expertise is thrust upon him.

Such a mindset can be very liberating for clients. Not infrequently, however, the client encounters it with incredulity and confusion.[3] He has come to the counselor's office as someone who is supposedly helpless, as someone who feels at the mercy of the problem. He experiences himself as suffering, marginalized, ignorant, and incapable. Moreover, now he is treated as an expert. This is surprising in any case. He was not prepared for this when he reported for consultation or received the invitation to a counseling session. Being confronted with one's own expert status for the first time in a consultation situation takes some getting used to. Thus, part of the counseling work consists of the client learning to perceive and value his competencies.

When a person seeking advice who has brought up a problem situation remembers, for example, because of an exception question, that she once successfully handled a similar situation, she often reacts with astonishment and relief. The facial features relax, a glow perhaps lights up the face, and the posture becomes more relaxed. Not infrequently, however, this astonishment is mixed with incredulity or even a dose of defensiveness: at that time, the situation was clearly different, the people involved were more benevolent, or she had simply been lucky.

With Milton Erickson (in Bamberger, 1999, p.22), it may be assumed that "there is no person who ever knows his true abilities." To be an expert on one's own life is therefore always a bit of an imposition. From this attitude, clients are approached as persons capable of making their own decisions. Furthermore, even if this is what they are looking for, it is, in many situations, not easy to bear. One's own maturity means, in any case, responsibility in the sense of self-responsibility. This responsibility can often not be taken on to its full extent without further thought, so that, for some time, guidance and support are necessary.

In principle, therefore, the Focus on Solutions approach treats clients as doers rather than victims, even though such a phrasing may reach its limits in certain circumstances. The idea of being a doer and shaper of one's life can be difficult to bear for certain people for cultural, social, and individual reasons. This must be taken into account in counseling. In our culture, for example, we can think of certain forms of religiosity

3 This is another reason why solution orientation and art orientation complement each other well: in the artistic work, the client experiences his expertise first-hand.

in which suffering and problems are understood to be willed by God. In any case, the postulated self-responsibility reaches its limits in the case of children, the very elderly, and those with certain disabilities.

For the counselor, too, an attitude that makes the client an expert is not easy to live with. Not only is he faced with the task of constantly observing this expertness, but he must also redefine the nature of his expertness. The traditional view, according to which the counselor, as an expert in problem-solving, has to find and implement solutions logically linked to the problem after an expert analysis of the problem, is no longer tenable. In the new view, he is neither an expert on problems nor solutions. He becomes an expert in the process that enables people to become clear about their goals, needs, resources, and abilities so that they can put this knowledge[4] to concrete use.

Metaphorically speaking, solutions are not generated in the counseling process or even delivered by the counselor but are already present in the client system beforehand. Thus, the professional counseling and therapy scenarios are about helping solutions to break through. Conversely, problems are not simply understood as obstacles but as a need for change or a necessity for it.

It should be relatively easy to concretize this new form of consulting expertise within the situation defined as supervision or coaching. Here, the counselor is not usually expected to know more or be able to do more than her client in all meaningful aspects. On the other hand, it is expected that she can use and promote existing possibilities and resources and can support the process in such a way that the expected success occurs.

It is much more unusual and therefore probably also more difficult to implement the client's expertise in counseling situations that are traditionally very hierarchically structured—as can be found to some extent in medicine, pastoral care, and management discussions—or where the client is in a situation that indirectly calls on the counselor

4 The inclusion of artistic expression and play—as is typical for Intermodal Decentering—makes it clear that this is not simply about rational, cognitive "knowledge" in the traditional sense, but about other forms of knowledge (physical knowledge, sensory knowledge, etc.), the perception and inclusion of which are just as important or even more important in certain situations and with certain people.

to "take charge" himself. This is especially true of young or particularly old clients, the severely disabled, and addicts. If professionals succeed in finding appropriate forms here as well, impressive successes are often reported.

Here we come up against the limits of a basic counseling attitude based on the client's expertise. In one case, there are limits of a cultural and institutional nature, which could be softened to the advantage of all involved. In the second case, limits of the client's physical, psychological, and spiritual capacity are in the foreground, and require appropriate adaptations from the counselor.

Problems are not rigidly coupled with solutions

In the first publications by de Shazer and his team that were translated into German, this basic assumption caused quite a stir. It contradicts the traditional view that only approaches specifically tailored to the problem can bring lasting success. For this reason, a great deal of diagnostic effort is expended in individual consulting sectors. The prevailing opinion there is that an appropriate, tailor-made solution can only be worked out after a detailed assessment of the problem situation.

De Shazer, in contrast, has shown that solutions are often structured much more simply than the problem. Daily consulting experience confirms this. However, de Shazer's wording can be misunderstood. The Focus on Solutions approach to work is not looking for a specific, simple solution that will eliminate the problem once and for all. Instead, it is about interventions that stimulate the client to take initial steps that lead towards a solution and, ultimately, a situation in which the problem no longer exists. It is about initiating a sustainable solution process. If this succeeds—that is, if a first perhaps small or perhaps surprisingly large success is achieved through a first step—the process often continues on its own and only needs to be accompanied and supported in a confirming manner. This continues until the problem has become irrelevant or is such that it can be well tolerated. However, if the conditions in the situation are unfavorable or if the client's self-esteem is severely impaired, the solution process requires more intensive, possibly long-term support from a professional.

The professional's initial solution-focusing interventions may seem unusual and simple to outsiders, but they are by no means easy to implement in the specific situation. Even the client's behavioral or attitudinal change, which marks the first sustainable step towards a solution, often seems surprisingly simple. Sometimes it can then be observed that the relief and success of this first step lead to a series of further behavioral and attitudinal changes that one would hardly have thought possible at the beginning. It is as if a "virtuous circle"—the opposite of the "vicious circle"—has been set in motion. In such cases, therapy or counseling can usually be completed after just two or three sessions, and follow-up checks show that the changes are lasting. The Focus on Solutions approach to work was often called "*Kurztherapie*" (short therapy) in the first decades because of such progressions.

Geared towards the future

The Focus on Solutions approach emphasizes a person's future orientation, focusing on a desired, positively imagined future. This does not mean negating the significance of the past or the importance of what is happening right now. But here, too, the focus is on resources. The successes or partial successes of the past are inquired about and highlighted. These are unique or rare exceptions within problematic states, strengths, and abilities that have received little attention so far or that have just become visible in the counseling situation.

The things to come are emphasized because a future that is described as concretely as possible and worth striving for is a strong driving force for someone to dare to take conscious steps into something new. The conversation itself takes a different turn. It moves out of the area of pathology, suffering, and problems and into the area of possible solutions.

Many clients' ideas about the future are vague, general, and imprecise. In difficult life situations, people sometimes forbid themselves to even think about a desirable future. For other clients, it is very unfamiliar to fantasize about something that may or may not come true. In counseling, it is therefore important to stimulate steps towards an imagined future in an animating but cautious and appreciative way. And, above all, to articulate these imaginings as concretely as possible or to express them artistically.

In talking about the future, we move into the world of the imagination or, as it is called in the age of the computer, the virtual. This can be pleasurable but also frightening. The counselor who himself enjoys the imaginative and at the same time adapts himself very precisely and appreciatively to the client's possible reactions will probably have the best chance of opening up the power of positive visions to his client.

The de Shazer approach is based on the observation that a concrete change in behavior is a great reality-shaping force, but only if it is associated with a corresponding change in meaning. This attention to behavior is accompanied by a preference for experiments, which represent tentative steps toward a new future.

"Would you be willing to go on a little experiment?" This or a similar question is asked in the central part of a counseling session, at which point the experiment envisioned is immediately carried out. The question can also be asked at the end of a counseling session, and the client is given finding the answer as a kind of homework assignment.

Engaging in experimentation is also typical of art-oriented work, which once again points to a certain inner kinship between these two approaches.

Clients want to cooperate—resistance does not exist

When, in 1984, after two years of back and forth, de Shazer was able to publish his essay on the "death of resistance" in the well-known American journal *Family Process* (de Shazer, 1984), he stirred up a lot of dust with this assertion. He argued that the concept of resistance, which has a specific place within the psychoanalytic theoretical model, is a bad idea that detracts from, rather than promotes, the effectiveness of therapeutic action. The concept of "resistance" was born in the brains of therapists but is now treated as a fact in practice. One cannot only blame the client for ineffective therapeutic treatment. Within systemic thinking, therapy is always a two-way process. For example, if family members do not complete a therapeutic task, they are not simply recalcitrant but are reacting to something the therapist has done or failed to do.

The Milwaukee Group substitutes the concept of *cooperation* for the concept of resistance:

> Each family, individual, or couple exhibits a unique way of cooperating, and the therapist's task is first to describe to himself or herself

> this specific way that the family exhibits and then to cooperate with it and in this way promote change. (de Shazer, 1989b, p.105)

Accordingly, the professional counselor's task is to develop the fit anew with each client system.

The Focus on Solutions approach accordingly advocates taking clients' desire to change at face value. In this context, change is understood as a continuous process of every human life and not as a (one-time or multiple) event.

Focus on Solutions also emphasizes relationship building, as highlighted earlier. It is underpinned by a fundamental appreciation of the other person, demands genuineness from the counselor, and must be open and clear. Furthermore, from our perspective, it requires the willingness to be "met" by the other person. According to Buber (1962), such a collision with the other person opens up the dimension of encounter. Encounter is not something purposeful. It has much to do with the phenomenon of being directly touched, which opens up and creates space, always for both client and counselor.

The significance and concretization of this form of professional relationship building are presented in detail in the textbook by Bürgi and Eberhart (2004).

A POSSIBLE MISUNDERSTANDING: NOT ALL SOLUTIONS ARE EQUAL

In the years before the turn of the millennium and the first years after, the word "solution" was, and still is, booming. Especially in politics and management, the expression is used very often. "We need solutions!" "We need to bring this issue to a solution!" The "solution orientation" is occasionally invoked in a way as if the very use of the expression guarantees that everything will change for the better.

Behind this use of the word, there is usually a way of thinking that in many respects contradicts the thinking presented in this book. Often, "solution" is used when one already has precise presuppositions about how this solution must be designed: it should meet these criteria or serve those interests. Occasionally, the opinion seems to prevail that there is only one solution to the problem, or the "ideal" solution is sought. Moreover, almost always, the opinion prevails that solutions can be worked out by a goal-oriented, rational, and linear procedure.

When we speak of a solution here, we have different notions. First, we use the word "solution" in a naive, unbiased way. We use the term when the problem that was brought into counseling no longer exists or has become so incidental, insignificant, or commonplace that it is perceived by those involved as an inconvenience or a peculiarity at most, but no longer as a problem. Second, we never start from the assumption that we have to look for a single, ideal solution. We have seen from experience that a wide variety of changes at very different levels can make a problem disappear. And third—and this is probably the most important and for many counselors the most unfamiliar thing—we have learned that many solutions come as a surprise.

What turns out to be a solution is often unexpected for the counselor or the client or both, not anticipated, and certainly not worked out step by step. This does not mean that a solution cannot be worked out in a consulting situation and derived quasi-logically from certain data. Such a path is undoubtedly feasible. However, this has often been tried in vain by the client himself or in cooperation with other counselors. Surprisingly, in Focus on Solutions consulting work and especially in Intermodal Decentering, something turns out to be a solution that was not previously considered at all.

The narrative approach according to Michael White

When people give accounts of themselves and their problems, they usually do so in the form of stories. For the narrative approach, introduced to us through the work of White and Epston (e.g., 1990), these stories, and thus the temporal and contextual dimensions of the problem presented, are in the foreground. Drawing on the thinking and research of Bateson (1981), arguably the most influential early thinker of systems theory directions within psychotherapy, Michael White, in the late 1980s, began to pay greater attention to the stories his clients reported to him.

It quickly became apparent that client stories are characterized by different themes. In one story, the theme of "loss" may predominate; in another, the theme of "insecurity" or "fear"; a third is shaped as a tragedy, etc. Simultaneously, it became clear that the nature of the theme very much influences what the corresponding client describes as currently problematic. White began to explore this phenomenon as well as other elements of the narratives presented.

"Good" client stories that engage the listener not only contain the events or the actions in their context, but they also elaborate the meanings attributed to the events and actions, and they spread out the ideas, thoughts, and images that the narrator has of himself and the world.

White's observations now showed that people who seek therapeutic or counseling help often have limited or poor stories. In extreme cases, such a client story is more or less reduced to a single, internalized diagnosis. "I'm depressed." "I'm just an alcoholic." The fact that the person in question is, for example, prudently and carefully tending a vegetable garden alongside his depression, or lovingly and faithfully caring for a grandchild as an alcoholic, is "forgotten," not mentioned, not in the person's field of vision. This is true not only for people who are labeled with a diagnosis but also for residents of shelters and homes for the elderly, for inmates of prisons and psychiatric clinics, and, in some cases, their relatives, as well as for members of social groups that have no voice in society—AIDS patients, the disabled, minorities, and so on. In terms of content, it also became apparent that people with mental health problems usually describe themselves very negatively in their stories. They are worthless, perhaps stupid, and "deserve" to have it bad. Positively valued skills and traits are almost completely absent.

White's therapeutic and counseling work is about engaging clients in conversations that bring out positive, buried, or neglected aspects of their lives and helping them to incorporate these into a new, less problem-saturated life story. In this way, the counselor becomes the co-author of an alternative story that is much richer than the original one and also contains positive aspects, opening up new possibilities. Through his questions, the therapist aims to help the client find content that can form a toolkit for building a new story. If this succeeds, it is a matter of anchoring the new story in the client's self-image on the one hand and making it known and spreading it in his social context on the other.

Accordingly, the narrative approach focuses less on clients' visions of goals and concrete behavior and more on the meanings that their experiences and behavior have for them. Meaning and sense-making are in the foreground. Meanings that people attach to their experiences are usually themselves wrapped up in stories. Counseling and therapy are about helping clients to have alternative stories and to have these stories heard in their immediate environments.

With such an approach, the narrative way of working is clearly on the ground of social constructivism. People live in a world of meanings. In the philosophical sense, this world is a constructed world. It becomes visible in the most diverse forms of human expression, but primarily in language. In everyday life, narrative language—in contrast to scientific language, for example—is in the foreground. This opens up a window to the human environment, to culture and society, but also to art in general and to poetry in particular.

The narrative approach can therefore also be understood as a literary approach.

Later, White (e.g., 2000) also emphasized social and societal concerns more and more. It was important to him to give a voice again to people who were not heard in society. He spoke of "re-membering" in contrast to the previous social exclusion of that member ("dismembering of a person's life"). Using the metaphor of an association or club ("a club of life"), he encouraged his clients to reconsider memberships in "their own club of life." As in other clubs, new members can be admitted, old memberships can be dissolved, honorary members can be appointed, or the previous membership of certain individuals can be suspended for a period of time. White's case reports show that this metaphor is very useful in helping people regain more agency in their self-image and in their actual lives (White, 1997, p.22).

A look at the methodical approach of Focus on Solutions

If, for the purpose of a summary, we take a look at behavioral or narrative Focus on Solutions work, the following can be seen.

In the consulting-therapeutic activity, the focus:

- is on what can be observed and concretely reported. Generalizing, abstract statements of the client are traced back to concrete experiences through questions. Everything that can be concretely observed in the session is used
- lies on the now and the future
- is based on what can be changed—i.e., scope for action, scope for thinking, scope for feeling are in the foreground

- focuses on what the client himself can change
- addresses the client as an active agent
- focuses on strengths and resources and on what has been achieved
- lies in the potentials and possibilities that can be discovered within the situation.

Theoretical backgrounds

SYSTEMS THEORY

The Focus on Solutions approaches were developed on the foundation of systems theory. This metatheory, which has received increasing attention within psychology and clinical practice since the second half of the last century, focuses not on exploring individual parts or aspects but on exploring the connections between the parts and describing and exploring the structures and processes that emerge from them. It cultivates, then, within the possible, a holistic view of phenomena, including the observer himself.

In particular, the last aspect had far-reaching consequences for therapeutic-counseling practice. If one understands the counseling setting as a system, the counselor can no longer make seemingly objective statements about the client or the events from a distance or intervene independently. All connections, including those between the observer and the observed person, must be understood as interrelationships with feedback processes. This recursivity in everything that happens emphasizes the processuality in action and the perspectivity of every statement in observation.

Based on systems theory, a linear cause–effect relationship is inconceivable. It is always and in every case about a reciprocal happening, even if one side of the influence may be incomparably stronger than the other. This is one reason why research into causes has a relatively low priority in forms of therapy based on systems theory. There is little search for causes or culprits. Instead, the nature, the organization of the connections, and their effects move into the foreground of attention.

Kriz (e.g., 1997a, 1997b, 2006) and others have linked systemic considerations with research results from chaos theory and synergetics. This has, among other things, brought phenomena of order and self-organization into focus. We have discussed these ideas in more detail earlier (see Section 6.3), as they seem helpful for understanding the processes we observe in Intermodal Decentering.

HUMANISTIC PSYCHOLOGY

In our understanding of Focus on Solutions practice, the body of thought of humanistic psychology plays a significant role. In German-speaking areas, this body of thought has been disseminated, for example, through the complete works of Carl Rogers (e.g., 1977) and those of Virginia Satir (e.g., 1975). Both authors emphasize that the resources for solutions lie in the person or in the corresponding social system itself.

Based on humanism and existential philosophy, the approaches of humanistic psychology emphasize above all the professional attitude and the connection between the professional as a person and the client.

Rogers and his person-centered psychotherapy focused on the process of becoming a person. This requires from the professional both a process-oriented approach and an encounter engagement that approximates the "I–Thou" connection described by Buber (Buber, 1962; Bürgi and Eberhart, 2004). Based on his conception of the human being and the results of his research on the therapy process, Rogers places particular emphasis on the attitude of the professional person observable in the conversational situation and here again on aspects such as authenticity, congruence, empathy, warmth, and (unconditional) attentiveness.

For her part, Virginia Satir, who worked primarily with families and couples, emphasizes the importance of supporting factors such as wholeness, growth, and self-worth.

The "idea of man" (*Menschenbild*) of humanistic psychology and its reflections on professional attitude and connection is an essential basis of our work and—from our point of view—central to Focus on Solutions in general.

SOCIAL CONSTRUCTIVISM

Epistemologically, Focus on Solutions is based on a constructivist view of human life: not only are statements about the objects we encounter in the world outside dependent on the location of the observer, but the neurophysiological processes we call perception literally construct them and do not merely map them, as we usually erroneously assume. This statement applies to perceptions but also to the products of thought or a feeling in response to an experience. In other words, there is theoretically an unlimited number of descriptions and explanations for every state of affairs. Heinz von Foerster (e.g., Foerster and Pörsken, 2004) therefore postulates: "The world is not found, but invented" ("*Die Welt wird nicht gefunden, sondern erfunden*") (1981 in Böse and Schiepek, 1989).

Human knowledge of the world and of ourselves is the result of construction processes. Contrary to statements of radical constructivism, the possibilities for descriptions and explanations are not unlimited. The way we describe, explain, and represent is influenced by our family background, our culture, the context in which we live, and thus ultimately derives from our relationships. Knowledge and experience, including scientific knowledge, are socially embedded—that is, culture-dependent. This is roughly the position of social constructivism, that relationships are the basis for everything that is understandable. Of course, it is true that every understanding of relationship is, in turn, shaped by culture and history. A statement receives the predicate "true" or "real" if it is shared by the group of significant people in the environment. This group, in turn, is embedded in the larger units of society and culture and their "truths." True, like good, depends on a continuous process of shared production of meaning and significance (Gergen, 2002). Thus, dialogue is of central importance in the construction of our world.

Social constructivism is "ontologically mute" (Gergen, 2002)—that is, it makes no statements about the nature of things. Nor does it destroy the ideas of truth, objectivity, science, morality, etc. What is called into question is the way in which these concepts have been understood and put into practice (Gergen, 2002, p.49).

If we transfer this understanding of the world and reality to the situation of counseling and therapy, it quickly becomes clear how significant this is. In the setting of counseling or therapy, embedded in a supportive relationship, there is a chance to create a (new) reality.

The forms of discourse in counseling and how we describe, explain, and interpret events change our view and our patterns of action. "In the way we enter into relationship with each other, we also construct our future" (Gergen, 2002, p.10).

It is evident that language, as well as other forms of communication, plays a central role in this. Modern Western man has developed something like a correspondence theory of language, assuming that words correspond to experienced realities. In contrast, social constructivism points out that language does not so much represent reality as create reality.

Therefore, if we begin, for example, in therapeutic dialogue, to express things language-wise in a different way for once, there is great power in this. "Through the power of language, new and different things can be made possible and given meaning. We come to this realization, however, only when we expand our repertoire of alternative descriptions and stop searching for the one, only true description" (Rorty, 1992, in Gergen, 2002, p.84). Language in this sense becomes something like social action or, to put it another way, a performance that involves constructing a (shared) world. This is also likely to apply unreservedly to shared artistic or playful activity. With this, the focus is placed on engaging with one another, being with one another, and doing with one another—in short, on the process.

The atmosphere of dialogue, the power of meaning-making that lies primarily in mutual affirmation, an unwavering belief in the client's unused or underused abilities, and an attentional focus on alternative voices, possibilities, and perspectives make social constructivism an excellent philosophical basis for therapeutic or counseling activity that produces lasting effects.

The significance of the imagination

In almost all psychotherapies known to us, dealing with imagination plays a significant role. Luc Ciompi (1982) has pointed out that the degree of freedom for a person in action is smaller than in emotional experience, and this, in turn, is smaller than in abstract-logical thinking. A philosopher, for example, who develops abstract thoughts, thus has the greatest degree of freedom, the greatest possibilities for play.

Ciompi did not mention the imagination, the mental doing-as-if, nor pictorial or aural imaginings, all of which also involve emotionality. It can be assumed that their degree of freedom would have to be classified somewhere between emotionality and abstract thinking.

A large degree of freedom makes it easier for people to change perspectives. It supports the flow of ideas and the emergence of new content.

The sustainable impact of the imagined "products" is more critical. They are somehow "airy" and can easily be "blown away by the wind." We can become aware of this very quickly when we think of the many resolutions we have already made but have not realized or have not realized for a long time. Nevertheless, it is true that many changes begin in the mind—that is, with the imagination of the desired future—or, as one would perhaps have to say today, first arise in the realm of the virtual. The lasting effect of such imaginings can be strengthened if it is possible to combine them with sensorial experiences, strong feelings, or motor activity—that is, with changed behavior.

Social constructionist considerations point out that changes are always connected with new meaning, new sense-making, indeed that the sense-making perhaps constitutes the sustainability of a change. Michael White would add that the new thing must be anchored in the self-image of the person concerned and, in addition, must be passed on, spread in the close social environment of the person concerned, if there is to be a guarantee that it will actually become part of the life concerned.

The imagination plays a vital role in Focus on Solutions work. This can be seen in the strong emphasis on imaginings, reflections, and fantasies about a future in which the problem no longer exists. It is also evident in the general use of language, in which the conditional form is very often used ("What if you made this new attitude more visible?"). Other question forms typical of Focus on Solutions counseling also make use of imagination. One can think of scaling questions or questions that include the external perspective ("If your wife were there, what would she say?").

8.4 Focus on Solutions and its criticism of other methods

People need patterns of order to deal with the world and the large number of impressions. These are patterns of action, patterns of thought, and patterns of emotional reactions. This statement is valid for the individual human being in everyday life and for his handling of problems. It also applies to science and religion.

Every pattern runs the risk of becoming absolutized and rigid. Absolutized patterns produce tyranny, rigid "law and order" situations, or fundamentalism. Rigid patterns are a basis on which pathology and destruction thrive.

Based on its conviction that perspectives other than the usual ones are possible in every situation, Focus on Solutions explicitly or implicitly relativizes and criticizes procedures that focus on an unquestionable "scientificity" of their approach.

The theoretical basis of systems theory and constructivism opens the Focus on Solutions approach to a diversity of perspectives. Systems theory also guards against using so-called "typical" Focus on Solutions questions as a method in a recipe-like manner. In contrast, the basic attitude of the professional person and her flexibility in shaping the process is more critical. Thus, Focus on Solutions strongly criticizes standardized, engineer-like approaches. On the contrary, it emphasizes the importance of surprises and strives to be attentive to them.

Structuralism, dominant in the social sciences and medicine in the Western world until recently, seeks the "actual" beneath or behind the surface of things. Therefore, counselors and therapists are urged not to be seduced by what is presented but to search "deeper."

The Focus on Solutions working approach criticizes this structuralist position, as is prevalent in many psychoanalytical approaches, for example. It is strongly oriented to what clients themselves present; it takes clients "at their word." It moves on the "surface" and strives for what is revealed to be presented in a phenomenological way as concretely and richly as possible.

This makes Focus on Solutions work very sensitive to language. In the verbal expression, the frame of thinking of the human being is revealed, or more generally and philosophically expressed: the nature of one's being-in-the-world. This criticizes the everyday behaviorist view that a problem is primarily about facts. From a Focus on Solutions perspective, it is not about the facts but about the meanings these facts have for a particular person.

The way a person expresses himself manifests the meanings he attaches to a thing, a person, or a circumstance. In the counseling situation, verbal expression plays a prominent role in addition to facial expressions and gestures. If one speaks in a different way about a known object, the connection between meaning and expression can now be used in the opposite way: "If I change the (verbal) expression, the meaning will change as well."

This connection is leveraged in the Focus on Solutions approach. By asking a client about new, unfamiliar aspects of a situation, the counselor elicits corresponding responses from the client. The meaning of the situation in question changes for the client.

This indirectly criticizes methods that bring to the fore the holistic experience of situations in the here and now. Focus on Solutions counters this view by saying that a change in verbal expression or, more generally, a change in behavior also changes the experience, which ultimately also changes what has been experienced as fact. This applies to the present and the future as well as to the past. The connection, however, is not a mechanical or linear one. The changed articulation triggers an irritation that has the potency to change the experiential quality of the memory, as well as the concrete experience. The nature of the change, however, cannot be directly influenced. If the quality of experience of a remembered, actual, or even expected event has changed, then in effect this event itself changes as well.

However, the most obvious and probably most important criticism is the view that in a problematic, difficult, or even pathological situation, the problem, difficulty, or pathology must be dealt with directly.

The fact that this attitude is so dominant and can be found almost everywhere is probably due not only to the underlying linear-mechanistic treatment logic (record and evaluate problem; determine cause(s); find corresponding antidote; use antidote and "finish" problem; conclude), but also to the fascination that something problematic exerts on almost all people. Problems are annoying, unpleasant, or disruptive. So what could be more obvious than to get rid of them as quickly as possible? However, problems can also be so oppressive and burdensome that they force people to deal with them intensively. And sometimes problems are so bizarre, strange, and incomprehensible that it is self-evident that dealing with them should be left to an expert. All this makes problems interesting and attractive, especially for people who are not directly affected by them.

The basic premise of Focus on Solutions is that the solution—or, rather, the solving—is independent of the problem. It is not the problem itself that needs to be addressed, but the exceptions and the client's strengths in general. This seems strange to many at first sight compared to what has been said above. And the conclusion from this—that the client is, in a certain sense, the expert in dealing with the problem—is unfamiliar and by no means attractive, especially for those who are in a difficult situation.

With this implication, Focus on Solutions criticizes the traditional medical approach. Traditionally, the counselor (medical doctor) sits in the expert chair: "After all, he has studied it." In the traditional medical model, which is by no means unique to medicine, the solution is sought outside the client and outside the relationship that has been established between the professional and the client. Either the solution sits in the mind of the counselor (e.g., in his experiences, his knowledge), or it sits in an abstract, higher-level system (e.g., in the science of the relevant field).

The disruption that Focus on Solutions makes in this regard is radical. It seeks the solution in the client, in her experiences, in her experience, and in her (fellow human) environment. And it shapes the counseling relationship in a way that solutions can show up.

In this context, the counselor's diagnostic efforts take on a new significance. A provisional process- and context-related diagnosis takes the place of an ascertaining and thus often fixing and labeling diagnosis. In many situations, such diagnoses could instead be called feedback. Feedback can be helpful, especially when given in the form of compliments. These are preferred in the Focus on Solutions approach. However, more important than all forms of diagnoses and feedback for Focus on Solutions is that something new is set in motion. It is towards this that the efforts of the professional person are directed.

9

Professional Requirements and Considerations on Continuing Education and Professional Development

9.1 Requirements for the counselor

Professional use of art and play

Our culture is inconceivable without manifestations of the artistic. Individuals today are more in touch with it than we often believe. To realize this, however, we must say goodbye to a classical ideal of education that places creative productivity at the center and not immediately disqualify the receptive attitude that is strongly evident today, for example, in the field of music and video, as an addiction to consumption. Those who work artistically with people today find time and again that a surprising ability to differentiate between the structure and content of a work of art can also develop through reception. People talk about their favorite texts, beautiful film scenes, and exciting developments in rap. They can not only name them but also describe them. This is true for all generations because they all increasingly have this access to the work of art. They differ only in their preferences regarding the style and genre of the artistic.

It is amazing how many people become productively artistic on their own initiative without having any professional aspirations. The young person who needs Photoshop software to create pictures is just as engaged as the retired person who is still beginning to learn how to yodel. We rarely find people in any social group or generation who are fundamentally opposed to this kind of relaxing or uplifting pleasure. If they are, they are mostly people who banish these activities tuned to the senses out of fundamentalist convictions.

The invitation to take up something artistic is usually not met with rejection by training participants. However, doubts often arise as to whether there are sufficient skills for a particular art discipline. A doubt can stem from a school situation where a clearly defined idea of the form and structure of the artistic product determined the aesthetics and thus also whether the product was right or wrong. For this reason, it is important as counselors to consistently adopt the solution- and resource-oriented attitude as we explained in Chapter 4 in relation to performance and aesthetics.

We draw on positive experiences in daily dealings with the artistic, find individual preferences, and emphasize playfulness. The first steps into artistic activity, which the layperson takes on her own initiative out of enthusiasm, are playful and unencumbered by the pressures of the art world. It is therefore essential to approach artistic activity in such a way that it is successful. For this, suitable activities are low-threshold in terms of manual dexterity but at the same time have high expressive power, as introduced under "low-skill–high-sensitivity" (see Section 4.6).

As we have seen, it is not necessary for the counselor or therapist to master all art disciplines, but she must have knowledge of the principles that govern an artistic process. Intermodal theory and the "low-skill–high-sensitivity" principle are helpful in guiding an artistic process in a medium outside one's own sensorial experience, the sensory-motivated creation, and the perception of the work process. The prerequisites for this are workshops on artistic craft, which are dedicated to this topic and encourage the participants to undertake their own experiments of artistic creation in our presence. Actually, the professional facilitators of change processes not only constantly practice counseling dialogue but also practice artistic experience as it can find space in our everyday culture. In this way, they increase the understanding of our contemporary art and, hopefully, its enjoyment, and they create a closer connection to cultural life.

Dealing with solution-oriented language and resource-oriented attitude

The principles of solution-oriented language, especially the typical question forms, are not difficult to learn. The logic behind the solution-oriented approach is also easy to understand. And yet, time and again, members of the helping professions have difficulty with it, both with solution orientation and with resource orientation. It is true what de Shazer has said again and again in his workshops: "it's simple but not easy"—that is, it is simple but it is not easy to deal with.

There are probably both cultural and individual reasons that resist the appropriation of the resource-oriented approach: on the one hand, the focus on successes or achievements contradicts both everyday behavior and Western consulting traditions. In wide circles of the population, it is still considered indecent to boast about one's successes (one's suffering, on the other hand, may, in most cases, be passed on without a second thought). Parents educate children and young people in this. Various sayings bear witness to this: "Pride comes before a fall," "*Nach em Lächli chunnt ds Bächli*" (Swiss German, meaning "If you flaunt your laughter too openly, tears will follow"). One fears the envy of others—or, as the Chinese say, the envy of the gods. However, one likes to deal with the problems, one's own and above all those of others, extensively and in public.

The Western counseling tradition is predominantly focused on the problematic, the suffering. If something is not going well, one has to deal with it in depth, as well as with the effects and causes. One must not "repress" it. Most of those seeking advice are of the same opinion. In the first session of counseling or therapy, they expect to be asked in detail about their suffering or inadequacy. Often there is also the hope that perhaps previously unknown reasons for the problem could be found in the counseling—apparently, on the assumption that one could then change something about the difficult situation sooner or with less effort.

This attitude and the assumptions behind it are not necessarily wrong. However, counselors and clients run the risk of falling into a form of problem trance together if they focus too intensively on suffering. Moreover, just as "solution language" creates a solution atmosphere, "problem language" can create a problem atmosphere in which everything looks even worse and more difficult than it already is.

Furthermore, a solution- and resource-oriented approach is also likely to threaten and challenge established positions of power. Those who seek help or ask for advice go to the expert as a person of authority who may be assumed to know more than they do. Whoever—conversely—sits in the counselor's or therapist's chair represents this authority, which is, moreover, in many places paired with the authority of the state. Institutions of psychiatry, social work or social pedagogy, school psychology, etc., come to mind. Working in these institutions provides the holders of the position in question not only with authority but also with security and support, which is associated with a certain power that is almost taken for granted.

The competence or maturity of the client, who is regarded as a "customer," contradicts this. It is therefore difficult to implement for professionals in these workplaces, especially because many clients do not perceive themselves as competent or knowledgeable, at least not in the context of the problem.

It is obvious: people who want to enter into a solution- and resource-oriented way of working have to relearn. This relearning concerns more the area of attitude than the area of practical process. The everyday life of education, further education, or professional development, which put the solution- and resource-oriented approach in the center, is complicated, for example, by the fact that many students already have years of experience in traditional helping professions. The focus on pathology, suffering, problems, or inadequacies has become second nature to them. Even if they are attracted by the new perspective and the new basic attitude, it takes a long time for the new to become something natural and then a habit.

9.2 Thoughts on continuing education and professional development

In general, basic training in the respective profession can and must be assumed for all professional facilitators of change processes. Psychologists, social workers, social pedagogues, members of teaching and healthcare professions, pastors, and other professions where person-to-person counseling or accompaniment is central come to mind. In the corresponding introductory training courses, usually designed as studies at universities, basic knowledge of psychology, psychopathology, and sociology and more or less rudimentary training in conversation and counseling are taught in addition to profession- and discipline-specific content.

In further education and professional development, however, there are always lateral entrants who want to professionalize themselves in counseling or accompanying work with people. They often have a lot of experience in a specific field of work—for example, as a volunteer—and have acquired a certain expertise in shorter or longer workshops and courses.

When we speak of *continuing education* below, we are not thinking of the introductory training courses mentioned above, but of postgraduate courses and comparable courses of study, usually lasting several years and usually part-time, in which the students are members of the professions mentioned above and have the relevant knowledge in addition to professional experience. If, for example, basic knowledge of interviewing is lacking, then this should be made up before the start of further training.

Professional development, in the terminology used here, is shorter programs, ranging from a two-day workshop to a series of two- to three-week courses.

The introduction to Intermodal Decentering within postgraduate studies

The difficulties faced by professionals who want to familiarize themselves with a solution- and resource-oriented way of working in an in-service postgraduate program lasting several years have already been described in Chapter 8.

To successfully overcome these difficulties, they must be addressed in the context of artistic empowerment. The merging of art-oriented and solution-oriented work is to be practiced throughout all courses. The art-analogous attitude, which sensitizes for the surprising, that which develops in the professional work of guidance, has its counterpart in the resource-oriented attitude. In this attitude, a "what else is" is always elicited from "what is." In this way, resources are brought into the light, which can have a very encouraging effect.

From the outset, in a comprehensive continuing education

program, artistic competencies must be approached in a resource-oriented manner and solution-oriented competencies in an art-analogous manner. If artistic competencies are approached in a deficit-oriented way, not only is the pedagogical approach contrary to the orientation of solution-oriented practice, but also the style of the artistic approach contradicts the practice of decentering. In such an approach, students would become aware of what they are not capable of while doing artistic work, which would completely contradict the decentering as a resource as we have described.

The situation is similar to the solution-oriented practice fields in continuing education. Here, the opportunity must be taken again and again to address learning difficulties or challenges by decentering. Here, too, a contradiction arises when difficulties in training deviate from the basic attitude that is being taught, and difficulties are thereby emphasized and problematized.

The objective of mutual interpenetration of competencies from the field of solution orientation and art orientation places a high demand on trainers. This not only requires didactics that approach the subject matter itself innovatively and are practiced in a "learning by doing" style, but also that artistic training should start in a solution-oriented way at the point where the participants currently come into contact with the artistic in their lives and are confronted with competency expectations in their work.

In conversation, the resulting aspirations are enriched. Among the visions that show up in connection with the arts, the frequency of "longing for beauty" is striking. As a consequence, the question of the outcome leads in each case to a training structure in the form of decentering, which then, in the aesthetic analysis, strengthens the perception for the creation and the process.

Finally, the harvest is, so to speak, the learning result.

In dance, for example, this can look like this:

> We are at the beginning of the course. We have noticed in conversation that an astonishing number of participants either occasionally dance to music by themselves at home or like to join in the ballroom (e.g., tango) or disco scene. Others like to go hiking or jogging, but all of them have the step in common with each other, which shapes

> the space or can be shaped by the space or the music as a path (or choreography). I am talking about contemporary dance theater, about Pina Bausch (Wuppertal Dance Theater) and her performance "Café Müller."[1]

This is an example of how stepping and a stage occupied with chairs can be used to create a "dance mobile" of an extraordinary kind, especially since the dancer (Pina Bausch) is sleepwalking and another dancer is constantly rearranging the chairs. I propose making an improvisation only with the simplest element, walking and stepping, and, in this way, pursue the idea that it is difficult to imagine dance without stepping. The teaching piece we are working on is called "Enter, Encounter." It connects to our situation. We enter the training, and we enter the encounter in dance with "low-skill–high-sensitivity."

This is already followed by sensitizing as a didactic element (SERA—see Section 4.6). We are at the edge of the studio and visually perceive the movement space, sensitize the body and breath while standing, and try to take the first step when it arises from the weight shift. The idea is to make it look like leaves coming off the tree, not regular, but creating tension for the audience ("When will the next leaf come? There's another one!"). The improvisation includes various spatial designs from the step. "How's it going?" (power, speed), "Where does it go?" (choreography), "How does it stand?" (silence); possibilities of meeting, going along, bouncing off, being in-between, what arises, chorus formation, etc.

Finally, an improvisation is worked out through various takes (i.e., new attempts). Aesthetic analysis trains the language of perception and process understanding of dance, which is different in each artistic discipline, even if they can be put into similar categories (see Chapter 4).

The situation in continuing education and training programs

Over the last decades, periodic professional in-service training has become commonplace among members of the psychosocial, medical, and educational professions. Within the quality management of

1 In the opening credits of the 2002 film *Hable con ella* ("Talk to her") by Pedro Almodóvar.

institutions and professional associations, this is a central concern. For professionals in whose daily work counseling, guiding, or therapeutic conversations occupy a central place, methodological training and continuing education are usually quite attractive, and this is what it is all about when someone wants to deal with the art- and solution-oriented approach.

In the following, we summarize our experiences in working with members of the professions mentioned, for whom Intermodal Decentering IDEC® is new. The situation presents itself differently in the related courses and workshops, depending on whether the focus is more on dealing with art or being resource-oriented and facilitating the conversation. Therefore, the situations that instructors face and the demands that are placed on them will first be described separately. Subsequently, we will then address some common aspects.

The (re)discovery of the artistic

For the vast majority of participants in training and continuing education, the artistic approach in a counseling situation is completely unfamiliar. However, as we have shown above in the professional approach to art and play, there are very rarely participants who are completely averse to the arts, as long as we take into account the entire spectrum of contemporary art, including music, print, and electronic media. We have also shown that many participants in continuing education courses are themselves involved in something artistically productive, be it tango dancing, Photoshop, or even in a music band.

For the hesitant among the students, who probably have access but do not trust themselves to create, we recommend that the assignment be carefully designed with "low-skill–high-sensitivity" in mind. The entry threshold must not be too high, nor should it arouse "old ghosts" from negative art education and ideas that grew out of it.

The confrontation with the process and resource orientation

The fact that the shaping of relationships plays a central role in success in counseling and therapy is part of the basic knowledge of the professional groups in question here (see also Bürgi and Eberhart, 2004, p.55). For most participants in our training and continuing education events, this is, therefore, a given. The specifics of the practical process, on the other hand, and especially the kind of relationship and attitude that is cultivated in the process- and resource-oriented work, can nevertheless cause difficulties.

Difficult for many is the change to a solution- and resource-oriented attitude. In short, professional development courses lasting only a few days, we have to take this very much into account. Our many years of experience in conducting training courses can be summarized as follows.

Anyone who has spent many years dealing in depth with the problems of his clients and has tried to grasp them in detail cannot expect to be able to switch to a solution-oriented approach and a resource-oriented attitude after a few days or weeks. A conversion period of one to two years is to be expected from personal experience and experience with participants in further education and training courses.

Reorientation is, of course, supported if the previously cultivated approach was either very laborious and time-consuming or often led to failure. However, in order to be ready for a change, in addition to concrete methodological instructions and plausible theoretical justifications, enough concrete examples are needed in which the positive effects of the solution-oriented approach become visible.

Examples have a motivating effect when they are made very concrete and easy to follow. This is why video recordings of counseling sessions in parts or as a whole usually have a better effect than written texts. Live demonstrations, in which both the client and the professional person have their say after the counseling session, have an even greater effect. Of course, this is only an option in coaching and supervision situations and not in a therapeutic situation.

We have had very good experiences with exercise settings in which course participants can experience the effect of a solution- and resource-oriented approach first-hand. We are not talking about role play here but about working on a personal concern in a solution-oriented way.

It is generally true that ingrained patterns of conversation cannot be successfully countered with arguments. Motivated by their own experiences and those of others, people are inspired to explore new ideas and earnestly learn and practice them based on an appreciation of the prior successes achieved with the method.

Once initial enthusiasm for the novel and unfamiliar approach has been generated, and the foundations for the methodological approach have been laid, the next step is to apply the new approach in one's own everyday practice, and not just once or twice on a trial basis, but again and again. The likelihood of this happening is reasonably assured if the institution or team in which the person in question works follows the same path. If this is not the case, it is highly recommended that a newly enthusiastic person joins forces with one or two like-minded people with a similar level of knowledge from other institutions and regularly exchanges experiences as well as celebrates the small and larger successes.

Equally challenging for many participants in further education and training courses is learning a counseling behavior that remains on the surface in conversation and in dealing with artistic activity and play. In the literature on solution-focused conversation, this is described as an attitude of not knowing. Epistemologically, we are in the field of phenomenology. This attitude of appreciative, curious openness, which is willing to take all statements of the person seeking advice at face value, for the time being, is a fundamental element of the solution- and resource-oriented attitude.

In terms of the method, the process-oriented approach must be practiced both in training courses and in advanced and further training, the approach that we have defined as "art-analogous." For many participants, this is also very unfamiliar and sometimes triggers apprehension, fear, and uncertainty. Our explanations, especially in Chapter 4, have shown that a session with an Intermodal Decentering phase is structured in a relatively simple and clear way. It is important, however, within this structure that the professional person initiates a process through questions and the shaping of the relationship and can then surrender to this process.

The professional person must learn to trust the process. This is not easy and may remain a lifelong task for many of us. First and foremost, it is about letting go of one's ideas about what should happen in the session in terms of content or what should be necessary for the client.

The process can therefore be best trusted by people who have experienced such processes, reflected on them, and experienced their good results. A suitable training vessel for such experiences is instructional supervision, instructional coaching, and instructional therapy.

In summary, it can be said that access to art and play is facilitated by the resource- and solution-oriented attitude. This happens to the same extent that artistic activity becomes a treasure trove for new aspects on the one hand and training for open, curious discovery on the other. This creates the conditions for a synergy of the two principles, which in turn stimulates and strengthens processes of self-organization. Training and further education must draw on this synergy and, as far as possible, avoid a mere stringing together of singular topics.

10

The Seriousness of Play and the Surprise of Art—Concluding Thoughts

We have chosen a philosophical title for our closing thoughts. It has something paradoxical about it. The seriousness is assigned to the play and the surprise to the art or the artistic work.

The title leads us once again to fundamental questions of the human encounter. Those who work with other people in a solution-oriented way and encourage and guide them from time to time to engage in an artistic work or a play remain very much committed to the concrete in their activities and are hardly tempted to reflect with clients on an abstract level in the course of counseling. The course of a session is characterized by a focus on the concrete, on the "surface" of statements and work. Nevertheless, it happens in our everyday counseling that philosophical questions about being human flow quite naturally.

On the one hand, this might have to do with the fact that we are open to metaphors that are expressed by the client and we work with them despite their lack of concreteness and rational indeterminacy.

Second, it should be remembered that in the harvesting phase, "second-degree solutions" often arise, which—from a different perspective—could be paraphrased as something like pearls of wisdom (see Section 4.8). It is not necessarily surprising, then, that conversations move on a philosophical level every now and then.

By being present in this way, we take the process of counseling very seriously, both as listeners and as speakers. The same applies when we guide an artistic process and are observers or participants in a play.

We have repeatedly pointed out the importance of this presence in the course of our discussion. It requires total commitment and a high degree of attention. This attention is not focused on specific content or behavior. Nevertheless, it is connected with an openness for what is revealed in the encounter, with a wide-angle view, so to speak, that is ready to take in everything that happens in the other person, in oneself, in the emerging work, in the play, and in the in-between.

With this openness and attention to the collaborative process and to what shows up in it as a surprise, commitment, presence, and seriousness are transformed. The personal commitment demanded of the professional person is at once engaging and relaxed. The presence demanded becomes a serene presence. And the seriousness becomes playful, comparable to the focused presence of a juggler or the seriousness of a toddler playing. Both give themselves fully to their play, always ready to react to what is surprising. Thus, in our approach, play and seriousness are intertwined in a distinct way.

Such an attitude has not only to do with lightness and a certain childlike impartiality, even though these descriptions may well apply. We do indeed try to approach what comes our way in clients' accounts and works with a certain lightness of touch. To the same extent, however, we take what is said and shown at its full face value and let ourselves be touched and seized by it. However, we do not take what is presented to us by the client as the only or final truth. On the contrary, we strive to allow other perspectives to appear as well, and we expose ourselves and our counterparts to the wealth of perspectives. We look for the exceptions behind or within the rule, even if this can sometimes have the effect of confusing the client.

Oddly enough, it is precisely this attitude and the resulting approach that very often open the door to fundamental aspects of being human and lead to conversations with philosophical or spiritual content. In this way, too, seriousness is involved in the play, a playing that we understand as "play" and not as "game." In earlier explanations, it was pointed out that this has a lot to do with the way we deal with art in Intermodal Decentering.

The connection between art and free play is close. Imagination plays a major role in both. In artistic activity, our work focuses on the unexpected and surprising. It can be observed in the work and the artistic process. In addition, in the artistic work, there is that which, simply put, confronts us as beauty.

It is about a broad, contemporary, and not a narrow, formal concept of beauty. It is about a sensorial phenomenon that occurs in the encounter that moves, touches, grips, and makes one marvel. It is something that opens our hearts in our work with people and their work. And it can get under the skin.

So it happens, then, that with our clients in the presence of the emerging work, a breath of beauty appears, in the face, in a movement, or in a spoken word.

Methodologically, our approach focuses on two aspects. First, it is what we call appreciative curiosity. This is an attitude that combines empathy with a spirit of inquiry and the joy of experimentation. It has an almost universally infectious effect on all participants and leads away from "right and wrong" to "let's see what it leads to."

Added to this is aesthetic responsibility. We understand this as being fully focused and present in the studio or workspace. Anything we undertake or direct in this area is done in the interest of the artistic process or toward the resulting work. That rules out choosing a medium or approach because it is likely to do the client good or might provide diagnostic clues.

And finally, one last thing. In writing this book, it has become increasingly clear to us that a core of our approach is a specific way of interweaving language and art. The art-analogous attitude in the encounter opens up the space of relationship and provides security. The solution-oriented dialogue and the attitude that goes with it give hope and bring about surprising enrichment. Furthermore, resource-oriented guiding in artistic activity allows works to flourish playfully into beauty.

In doing so, we touch on something that reaches beyond us, that was not there before, and that "speaks to us" or "tells us something." It is conceivable that for this reason, too, some people come to talk about questions of meaning on their own initiative or address spiritual issues in the course of the work. The pioneers of solution-focused conversation never sought such a thing. Nor was such a thing envisaged in the traditional approach to art in the practice fields of therapy and counseling, with their cathartic, educational, relaxing, or even diagnostic concerns.

The resource-oriented attitude, solution-oriented dialogue, and the openness and surprises of artistic activity have a stimulating and supportive effect on the forces of self-organization and self-healing; this, in turn, frees the individual to turn to the present and central aspects of shaping his or her life.

References

Anderson, H. and Goolishian, H.A. (1990) Menschliche Systeme als sprachliche Systeme. *Familiendynamik* 15 (3): 212–243.

Bamberger, G.G. (1999/2005) *Lösungsorientierte Beratung*. Weinheim.

Bateson, G. (1981) *Ökologie des Geistes. Anthropologische, psychologische, biologische und epistemologische Perspektiven*. Frankfurt a. M.

Baudelaire, C. (1923). *Tableaux parisiens*. Die Drucke des Argonautenkreises: Druck 5. Heidelberg: R. Weissbach.

Bengel, J., Strittmatter, R., and Willmann, H. (1998) *Was erhält gesund? Antonovskys Modell der Salutogenese. Diskussionsstand und Stellenwert. Eine Expertise*. Köln.

Benjamin, W. (2002). "The Task of the Translator" (Die Aufgabe des Übersetzers). In M. Bullock, & M. W. Jennings (Eds.), Walter Benjamin: Selected Writings. Volume I: 1913-1926 (pp. 253-263). Cambridge, MA: Harvard University Press.

Benjamin, W. (2002). "The Task of the Translator" (Die Aufgabe des Übersetzers). In M. Bullock, & M. W. Jennings (Eds.), Walter Benjamin: Selected Writings. Volume I: 1913-1926 (pp. 253-263). Cambridge, MA: Harvard University Press.

Böse, R. and Schiepek, G. (1989) *Systemische Theorie und Therapie. Ein Handwörterbuch*. Heidelberg.

Boss, M. (1982) *Psychoanalysis and Daseinsanalysis*. New York.

Brodbeck, K.-H. (1999) *Entscheidung zur Kreativität*. Darmstadt.

Bruner, J. (1986) *Actual Minds, Possible Worlds*. Cambridge.

Buber, M. (1962/1994). *Das dialogische Prinzip* (7. Auflage). Gerlingen.

Bürgi, A. and Eberhart, H. (2004) *Beratung als strukturierter und kreativer Prozess. Ein Lehrbuch für die ressourcenorientierte Praxis*. Göttingen.

Callahan, R.M. (1992) *Imagining Imagination: A Phenomenological Study of Children's Drawings of Imagination*. Dissertation, Cambridge, MA.

Cecchin, G., Lane, G., and Ray, W.A. (1993) *Respektlosigkeit. Eine Überlebensstrategie für Therapeuten*. Heidelberg.

Ciompi, L. (1982) *Affektlogik. Über die Struktur der Psyche und ihre Entwicklung. Ein Beitrag zur Schizophrenieforschung*. Stuttgart.

Decker-Voigt, H.-H. (ed.) (1983) *Lexikon der Musiktherapie*. Lilienthal/Bremen.

de Jong, P. and Berg, I.K. (1998) *Lösungen (er)finden. Das Werkstattbuch der lösungsorientierten Kurztherapie*. Dortmund.

de Shazer, S. (1984) The death of resistance. *Family Process 11* (1): 11–21.

de Shazer, S. (1989a) Der Dreh. Überraschende Wendungen und Lösungen in der Kurzzeittherapie. Heidelberg.

de Shazer, S. (1989b) *Wege der erfolgreichen Kurztherapie*. Stuttgart.

Dolan, Y.M. (1985) *A Path with a Heart. Ericksonian Utilization with Resistant and Chronic Clients*. New York.

Eberhart, H. (2004) Dezentrierung und Überraschung in der kunst- und ausdrucksorientierten Arbeit. In: H. Eberhart and H. Killias (eds) *Überraschung als Anstoss zu Wandlungsprozessen*. Zürich.

Eberhart, H. (ed.) (2007) *Kunst wirkt. Kunstorientierte Lösungsfindung in Beratung, Therapie und Bildung*. Zürich.

Eberhart, H., & Knill, P. J. (2010). *Lösungskunst: Lehrbuch der kunst- und ressourcenorientierten Arbeit ; mit zwei Tabellen* (2., erg. Aufl.). Göttingen: Vandenhoeck & Ruprecht.

Ellis, A. and Grieger, R. (eds) (1979) *Praxis der rational-emotiven Therapie*. München: Urban und Schwarzenberg.

Foerster, H. von and Pörksen, B. (2004) *Wahrheit ist die Erfinder eines Lügners*. Heidelberg.

Fuchs, M. (1994) *The Art of Structuring*. Lesley University, Cambridge, MA (unpublished handout).

Fuchs, M. (2002) Tiefe liegt auf der Hand oder von der Kunst, am Obergrund zu bleiben. In: S.K. Levine (ed.) *Crossing Boundaries. Explorations in Therapy and the Arts*. Toronto.

Fuchs, M. (1994) *The art of structuring*. Lesley University, Cambridge MA (unpublished handout).

Gadamer, H.-G. (1977) *Die Aktualität des Schönen*. Stuttgart.

Gardner, H. (1991) *The Unschooled Mind. How Children Think and How Schools Should Teach*. New York.

Gergen, K.J. (2002) *Konstruierte Wirklichkeiten. Eine Hinführung zum sozialen Konstruktionismus*. Stuttgart.

Gingerich, W.J. and de Shazer, S. (1991) The BRIEFER Project: Using expert systems as theory construction tools. *Family Process* 30 (2): 241–250.

Gronau, B., & Lagaay, A. (2010). Ökonomien der Zurückhaltung: Kulturelles Handeln zwischen Askese und Restriktion. Kultur- und Medientheorie. s.l.: transcript Verlag.

Grotowski, J. (1968/2002). *Towards a Poor Theater*. New York.

Haken, H. (1995). *Erfolgsgeheimnisse der Natur. Synergetik—Die Lehre vom Zusammenwirken*. Reinbek.

Haken, H. (2004) Ist der Mensch ein dynamisches System? In: A. von Schlippe and W.C. Kriz (eds) *Personzentrierung und Systemtheorie. Perspektiven für psychotherapeutisches Handeln*. Göttingen.

Haken, H. and Schiepek, G. (2006) *Synergetik in der Psychologie. Selbstorganisation verstehen und gestalten*. Göttingen.

Heidegger, M. (1960) *Der Ursprung des Kunstwerkes*. Stuttgart.

Husserl, E. (1952) *Ideen zu einer reinen Phänomenologie und phänomenologischen Philosophie. Gesammelte Werke, Band IV (aus dem Nachlass)*. Den Haag.

Jacoby, M. (2003) The poietic basis of being: Thoughts on expression and the other person. Based on the work of Merleau-Ponty. *Poiesis. Journal of the Arts & Communication* 5: 106–114.

Jennings, S. (1995) *Theater, Ritual and Transformation. The Senoi Temiars*. London/New York.

Kähler, H.D. (1991) *Erstgespräche in der sozialen Einzelhilfe*. Freiburg i. Br.

Kluge, F. (1975) *Etymologisches Wörterbuch*. Berlin.

Knill, P.J. (1979) *Ausdruckstherapie. Künstlerischer Ausdruck in Therapie und Erziehung als intermediale Methode*. Lilienthal/Bremen.

Knill, P. (1982) Strukturparallelen zwischen Musiktherapie und Spieltherapie. *Musiktherapeutische Umschau* 3: 1–8.

Knill, P.J. (1986). Theory indigenous to art. *Journal of the International Association for Art, Creativity and Therapy (IAAACT)* 3 (2).

Knill, P. (1990a) Gibt es eine "kunstgerechte" Forschung in der Kunsttherapie? *Forum für Kunsttherapie* 3 (2): 32–39.

Knill, P. (1990b) Das Kristallisationsprinzip in einer musikorientierten Psychotherapie. In I. Frohne (ed.) *Musik und Gestalt*. Paderborn.

Knill, P.J. (1995) Ist Schönheit bildend und heilsam? Eine Stellungnahme zur Ästhetik in der Kunstpädagogik. In: W. Schiementz and J. Beilharz (eds) *Ins Bild gesetzt. Facetten der Kunstpädagogik*. Weinheim.

Knill, P.J. (1999) Expressive Arts: The intermodal language of imagination. In: S. Levine and E. Levine (eds) *Foundation of Expressive Arts Therapies*. London.

Knill, P. (2002). Mannigfaltigkeit als Tradition. Theorien zu interdisziplinären Kunsttherapien. Ein Überblick. *Forum für Kunsttherapie* 15 (1): 37–49.

Knill, P.J. (2004) Chaos, Hoffnung und Kunst. In: A. von Schlippe and W. Kriz (eds) *Personzentrierung und Systemtheorie, Perspektiven für psychotherapeutisches Handeln*. Göttingen, S.

Knill, P.J., E.G. Levine, and S.K. Levine (2004) *Principles and Practice of Expressive Arts Therapy*. London.

Knill, Paolo (2007) "Community Art," die Kunst und das Gemeinwesen. In: H. Eberhart (ed.) *Kunst wirkt. Kunstorientierte Lösungsfindung in Beratung, Therapie und Bildung*. Zürich.

Knill, P.J., Barba, H., and Fuchs, M. (1993/1995) *Minstrels of Soul. Intermodal Expressive Therapy*. Toronto.

Krieger, D. (1997) *Kommunikationssystem Kunst*. Wien.

Kriz, J. (1997a) *Chaos, Angst und Ordnung*. Göttingen.

Kriz, J. (1997b) *Systemtheorie. Eine Einführung für Psychotherapeuten, Psychologen und Mediziner*. Wien.

Kriz, Jürgen (2002) Expressive Arts Therapy. Ein "Spiel-Raum" für mehr Spielraum in den Sinnstrukturen der Lebenswelt. In: S.K. Levine (ed.) *Crossing Boundaries. Explorations in Therapy and the Arts*. Toronto.

Kriz, J. (2004) Überraschung: Eine Botschaft der Ordnung aus dem Chaos. In: H. Eberhart and H. Killias (eds) *Überraschung als Anstoss zu Wandlungsprozessen*. Zürich.

Kriz, J. (2006) *Self-actualization*. Norderstedt.

Kriz, J. (2007) Zur Wirkungsweise der Kunst- und Ressourcenorientierten Arbeit. In: H. Eberhart (ed.), *Kunst wirkt. Kunstorientierte Lösungsfindung in Beratung, Therapie und Bildung*. Zürich.

Lahad, M. (1992) The Six Pieces Story Making. In: S. Jennings (ed.) *Dramatherapy. Theory and Practice*. London.

Langen, D. (1973) *Psychotherapie. Kompendium für Studierende und Ärzte* (3. *Auflage*). Stuttgart.

Lempert, T. (2007) Wenn das Rosa schmutzig bleibt. Ästhetische Verantwortung im kunsttherapeutischen Setting. In: H. Eberhart (ed.) *Kunst wirkt. Kunstorientierte Lösungsfindung in Beratung, Therapie und Bildung*. Zürich.

Levine, E. (1995) *Tending the Fire. Studies in Art, Therapy and Creativity*. Toronto.

Levine, S.K. (2002) Chaos and Order: Rudolph Arnheim's Gestalt Psychology of Art. *Gestalt Theory Jahrbuch*: 266–288.

Lorenz, K. (1987) *Die Rückseite des Spiegels*. München.

Lorenzer, A. (1984) *Intimität und soziales Leid. Archäologie der Psychoanalyse*. Frankfurt a. M.

Mastnak, W. (1993) Polyästhetische Erziehung und Tiefenpsychologie. In: W. Roscher (ed.) *Sinn und Widerspruch musikalischer Bildung. Beiträge zu "poiesis."* München/Salzburg.

Maturana, H.R. and F.J. Varela (1987) *Der Baum der Erkenntnis. Die biologischen Wurzeln menschlichen Erkennens*. Bern/München.

Mattmüller, F. (1979) *Miteinander lernen macht frei! Handbuch für einen lebendigen Unterricht*. Basel.

McNiff, S. (1981) *The Arts and Psychotherapy*. Springfield.

McNiff, S. (1988) *Fundamentals of Art Therapy*. Springfield.

McNiff, S. (1998) *Art-Based Research*. London.

Meier, G. (1988) *Am Anfang war das Wort*. Bern.

Merleau-Ponty, M. (2001) *Phenomenology of Perception*. London.

Merton, R.K. (1995) *Soziologische Theorie und soziale Struktur*. Berlin.

Metzger, W. (1962) *Schöpferische Freiheit*. Frankfurt a. M.

Mogel, H. (1990). *Psychologie des Kinderspiels* (2. Auflage). Berlin.

Moreno, J.L. (1967) *Die Grundlagen der Soziometrie*. Opladen u. Wiesbaden.

Pfeifer, W. (Ed.) (2010). *Etymologisches Wörterbuch des Deutschen*. Koblenz: Ed. Kramer im Rhenania-Buchversand.

Piaget, J. (1937/1998). *Der Aufbau der Wirklichkeit beim Kinde*. Stuttgart.

Rogers, C. (1974) *Lernen in Freiheit*. München.

Rogers, C. (1977) *Therapeut und Klient. Grundlagen der Gesprächspsychotherapie*. München.

Rorty, R. (1992) *Kontingenz, Ironie und Solidarität. zitiert nach Gergen, Kenneth J. (2002): Konstruierte Wirklichkeiten. Eine Hinführung zum sozialen Konstruktionismus*. Stuttgart.

Roscher, W. (1980) Polyästhetische Erziehung, in: *Musik und Bildung*, 12, 5, S. 318-319. Mainz: Schott Music Distribution.

Rosen, S. (1985) *Die Lehrgeschichten von Milton H. Erickson*. Hamburg.

Saß, H., Wittchen, H.-U., and Zaudig, M. (eds) (1996) *Diagnostisches und statistisches Manual Psychischer Störungen DSM-IV*. Göttingen.

Satir, V. (1975) *Selbstwert und Kommunikation. Familientherapie für Berater und zur Selbsthilfe*. München.

Schiepek, G., Eckert, H., and Weihrauch, S. (2005) Prozessmonitoring dynamischer Systeme. *Systeme* 19 (2): 177–209.

Schiffer, E. (2001) *Wie Gesundheit entsteht. Salutogenese: Schatzsuche statt Fehlerfahndung*. Weinheim.

Schleiermacher, F. (1838). Friedrich Schleiermacher's sämmtliche Werke. Berlin: Reimer.

Schlippe, A. von and Lob-Corzilius, T. (1993) Chronische Krankheit im Kontext der Familie. *Familiendynamik 18* (1): 37–55.

Schnebel, D. (1930) "Das Urteil" und "Glossalie" (zwei Kompositionen).

Schulte, R., & Biguenet, J. (Eds.) (1992). *Theories of translation: An anthology of essays from Dryden to Derrida*. Chicago: University of Chicago Press

Schwarzbauer, M. (ed.) (2001) *Polyästhetik und Bildung*. Frankfurt a. M.

Shazer, S. de (1982). *Patterns of brief family therapy: An ecosystemic approach*. The Guliford family therapy series. New York: Guilford Pr.

Simon, F.B. (1991) *Meine Psychose, mein Fahrrad und ich. Zur Selbstorganisation der Verrücktheit*. Heidelberg.

Steiner, T. and Berg, I.K. (2005) *Handbuch lösungsorientiertes Arbeiten mit Kindern*. Heidelberg.

Stierlin, H. (1990) Zwischen Sprachwagnis und Sprachwirrnis. *Familiendynamik* 15 (3): 266– 275.

Stige, B. (2001) Polyphonic Voices, Aesthetic Aspects of Music Therapy Improvisations. In: *Berufsverband der Musiktherapeutinnen und Musiktherapeuten in Deutschland e. V. (BVM): Einblicke. Beiträge zur Musiktherapie*. Vol. 12. Berlin.

Strunk, G. and Schiepek, G. (2006) *Systemische Psychologie. Eine Einführung in die komplexen Grundlagen menschlichen Verhaltens*. München.

Szeemann, H. (1983) *Der Hang zum Gesamtkunstwerk*. Aarau.

Tschacher, W. (2004). Kognitive Selbstorganisation als theoretische Grundlage eines personzentrierten Ansatzes. In A. von Schlippe and W.C. Kriz (eds) *Personzentrierung und Systemtheorie. Perspektiven für psychotherapeutisches Handeln*. Göttingen.

Tüpker, R. (1988) *Ich singe, was ich nicht sagen kann. Zu einer morphologischen Grundlegung der Musiktherapie*. Regensburg.

Watzlawick, P., Beavin, J.H., and Jackson, D.D. (1969) M*enschliche Kommunikation. Formen, Störungen, Paradoxien*. Bern.

White, M. (1989) *Selected Papers*. Adelaide.

White, M. (1997) *Narratives of Therapists' Lives*. Adelaide.

White, M. (2000) *Reflections on Narrative Practice*. Adelaide.

White, M. and Epston, D. (1990) *Die Zähmung der Monster. Literarische Mittel zu therapeutischen Zwecken*. Heidelberg.

Index

adolescents in counseling sessions 92
aesthetic analysis
  and artistic expression 186
  in counseling sessions 77, 81, 86–9, 118, 120, 132, 137, 141, 146, 147–8, 151, 152, 153, 154, 155–6, 160, 175–6, 199–200
  in group working 224, 226
  and imagination 188
  in Intermodal Decentering 220–1
  and language 185
  and play 189, 190
  and possibilities in artistic activities 30
  in professional development 283
  and substitution model 214–15
  and supervision 222
  and third party artistic activity 195–6
  in working with clients 50
analysis of counseling sessions 144–7
Anderson, H. 180, 182, 183
appreciative curiosity
  in counseling sessions 77–8, 96–7, 168–70
  of counselors 43
  description of 290
  and language 27, 183
  and transference 80
Arnheim, Rudolf 246
art-analog process in counseling 72–3
art-orientated practice 251–4
artistic expressions 44–5
  holistic view of 241–3
  and play 186–7
artistic activities
  attractiveness of 31
  body–soul dimension in 63–4
  decentering in 61–3, 70–2, 189–91
  enrichment with language 32–4
  intermedial transfer in 249
  interpersonal aspects of 248–9
  interventions in 65–6
  intrapersonal aspects of 249–50
  new possibilities through 27–31
  personal empowerment through 66–8
  professional use of 279–80
  and self-organizing 212–13
  as sense activity 31–2
  third-party 195–6
  transpersonal aspects of 250–1
assignments in counseling sessions
  adolescents in 92
  between sessions 170–3
  children in 92
  different approaches to 90–1
  and hidden assignments 93
  and mandated clients 91–2
  self-checking in 93–4
  and third-party assignments 92–3
  uncompleted 176–8
assistance in harvesting 156–7
association gathering in counseling sessions 157–8
attractiveness of artistic activities 31

Bamberger, G.G. 257, 260
Bateson, G. 256, 266
Baudelaire, C. 19
behavioral approach 255–7
Bengel, J. 216, 226
Benjamin, W. 19
Berg, I.K. 92, 99, 107, 174, 175, 257
Biguenet, J. 20
body–soul dimension in
artistic activities 63–4
Böse, R. 271
Boss, M. 58, 246
boundaries in counseling
sessions 104–6
bridging in counseling
sessions 117–20
Brodbeck, K.-H. 75
Bruner, J. 180
Buber, M. 76, 265, 270
Bürgi, A. 76, 180, 265, 270, 284

Callahan, R.M. 242
Cecchin, G. 76
children in counseling sessions 92
Ciompi, L. 272
clients
appreciation of 75–7
and cooperation 264–6
and counseling relationship 72–80
empowerment of 43–4
as experts 43, 259–62
and harvesting 164–5
mandated clients 92
and resource-oriented
approaches 43, 205
stories of 181–6
coaching in decentering 221–3
concerns in counseling sessions
boundaries in 104–6
centrality of 94–5
changes in emphasis 102–4
counselors view of 100–2
descriptions of 96
and empathy 95
exceptions in 99–100
and being good to self 100
paraphrasing 96–7
problem-free times 97–9
and problem trance 95–6
time limitations in 101–2
condition–consequence structure 46
counseling
appreciation of client 75–7
art-analog process in 72–3
and client relationship 72–80, 70
counselor as expert in 79
epistemological aspects of 69–70
imaginative spaces in 59–61
initial interviews 78–9
interdisciplinary approach to 64–5
listening in 74–5
Notenge in 57–61
openness in 74–5
and presence 75
rituals in 55–6
transference in 79–80
counseling sessions
assignment clarification in 89–94
bridging 117–20
concerns in 94–106
decentering in 82–9, 120–55,
159–61, 163–73, 198–9, 211–12
effects in 107–201
examples of 83–9, 102–4,
113–14, 143, 159–61, 163–4,
165–9, 171–4, 176, 177–8
good results in 106–17
and harvesting 154–70, 199
phases of 81–9
counselors *see* professionals
crystallization principle 245, 247–8
curiosity in counseling
sessions 168–70

decentering
as action 191–2
analysis and feedback 144–7
and artistic activities 61–3,
63–9, 189–91
coaching in 221–3
in counseling sessions 82–9,
120–55, 159–61, 163–73, 211–12
description of 27–8
and experiential content 151–2

and language 186
and limits 236–7
and low-skill-high-sensitivity activities 122–3
and play 63–9, 70–2, 188–91
process in 150–1
sensitivity and motivation raising 123–8
studio atmosphere enhancements 128–42
supervision in 221–3
and surface 147–50
and sustainability 201–5
theme near- and theme far- 142–4
Decker-Voigt, H.-H. 245
de Jong, P. 99, 107, 174, 175, 257
de Shazer, S. 94, 105, 107, 111, 174, 175, 176, 255, 256, 257, 262, 264–5, 279
Dolan, Y.M. 95

Eberhart, H. 21, 35, 76, 78, 180, 265, 270, 284
effects in counseling sessions
after conclusion of 199–201
in decentering phase 198
in first conversation phase 197–8
during harvesting 199
long-term effects 204
Ellis, A. 252
empathy in counseling sessions 95
enrichment in counseling sessions 174–5, 213–14
epistemological aspects of counseling 69–70
Epston, D. 99, 266
experiential content in decentering 151–2
expressions of good results in counseling sessions 113–15
expressiveness-oriented practice 251–4

feedback from counseling sessions 144–7
"fixed scripts" in language 26
Focus on Solutions practice 47, 48, 77, 99, 113, 254–76
Foerster, H. von 271
Fuchs, M. 21, 216, 239, 242, 246

Gadamer, H.-G. 45
Gardner, H. 40
Gergen, K.J. 69, 196, 271, 272
Gingerich, W.J. 256
good results
ambivalence of 115–16
details of 108–10
imagining 107–8
expansion of 113
expressions of 113–15
language in 112–13
professional view of 106–7
questions of 111–12
time horizons for 110–11
and utopian goals 116–17
Goolishian, H.A. 180, 182, 183
Grieger, R. 252
Gronau, B. 20
Grotowski, J. 121, 246
group working 223–6

Haken, H. 73, 193, 206, 208
harvesting
and aesthetic analysis 175–6
and assignments 170–3, 176–8
assistance in 156–7
client participation in 164–5
counselor participation in 158–62
curiosity in 168–70
description of 154
effects in 199
and enrichment 174–5
gathering associations 157–8
initial questions 155–6
integration stage in 163–4
next step discussions 165–8
and solutions of the second order 162–3
Heidegger, M. 45, 77
hidden assignments 93
holistic view in art therapies 239–47

humanistic psychology 270
Husserl, E. 194

imagination
and aesthetic analysis 188
in art and play 289–90
imagining good results 107–8
and Intermodal Decentering 244–5
significance of 272–3
imaginative spaces in counseling 59–61
initial interviews 78–9
initial questions 155–6
interdisciplinary approach to counseling 64–5
intermedial transfer in artistic activities 249
Intermodal Decentering
counselors use of 49
and crystallization principle 245, 247–8
description of 28
as hybrid 47–8
and imagination 244–5
limits of 235–6
and methodological approach 33–4
not knowing in 77
in therapy 219–21
interpersonal aspects of artistic activities 248–9
interventions in artistic activities 65–6
intrapersonal aspects of artistic activities 249–50

Jacoby, M. 70
Jennings, S. 122

Kähler, H.D. 92
Kluge, F. 187
Knill, P.J. 11, 12, 13, 14, 21, 22–3, 35–6, 68, 72, 78, 123, 130, 144, 145, 187, 206, 225, 239, 242, 245, 246, 247, 248, 252
Krieger, D. 45
Kriz, J. 22, 25, 32, 69, 72, 82, 193, 206, 207, 209, 211, 212, 213, 269

Lagaay, A. 20
Lahad, M. 218
Langen, D. 46
language
and client stories 181–6
counselors use of 179–80
enrichment of 27
enrichment with artistic activities 32–4
"fixed scripts" in 26
focus on 196–7
and Focus on Solutions 274–5
and good results in counseling sessions 112–13
new realities through 180
psychologists use of 25
and substitution model 215–16
Lempert, T. 220
"less is more" instructions 130–2
Levine, E. 22, 105
Levine, S.K. 22, 246
limits
of decentering 236–7
of Intermodal Decentering 235–6
psychological danger as 233–4
unstable situations 234–5
listening in counseling 74–5
Lob-Corzilius, T. 181
Lorenz, K. 187
Lorenzer, A. 254, 255
low-skill-high-sensitivity activities
in counseling sessions 122–3, 138, 139, 144
in decentering 190
in holistic view of art therapies 245
and professional development 278, 283, 284
and psychological danger as limit 233
and solution-orientated approaches 40–1

Mastnak, W. 245
Maturana, H.R. 209
Mattmüller, F. 40
McNiff, S. 133, 242, 246, 253
Meier, G. 188
Merleau-Ponty, M. 21, 45, 70–1
Merton, R.K. 108
metacommunication in counseling 79
Metzger, W. 206–7
Mogel, H. 131
Moreno, J.L. 240, 241, 248
motivation raising in counseling sessions 123–8

narrative approach 266–8
not knowing in counseling 77–8
Notenge
 in counseling 57–61
 and decentering 62
 as problem 94

openness in counseling 74–5
order, problem with 206–7

Pfeifer, W. 22
phases of counseling sessions 81–9
phenomenological approach 44, 194–5, 196
Piaget, J. 130, 206, 245
play
 and artistic expression 186–7
 categories of 187–9
 decentering in 63–9, 70–2, 188–91
 description of 187–8
 expansions of 68–9
 professional use of 279–80
polyaesthetics 245
Pörksen, B. 271
presence in counseling 75
problem-free times in counselling sessions 97–9
problem trance 95–6
process in decentering 150–1
professionals
 appreciative curiosity of 43
 art and play use by 277–8
 and concerns in counseling sessions 100–2
 continuing development for 281–7
 and good results in counseling sessions 106–7
 and harvesting in counseling sessions 158–62
 phenomenological attitude of 44
 postgraduate study of 281–3
 working with clients 48–54
psychologists
 language use 25

Reich, Wilhelm 240
resource-oriented approaches
 and artistic activities 253
 changes through 42
 in counselling sessions 150, 152, 174
 and decentering 204, 212
 enrichment with artistic activities 33
 and expression 44
 and Focus on Solutions 256–7
 and good futures 47, 116
 and language 183
 and Intermodal Decentering 219, 221, 281, 282, 235
 and multisensory approach 12
 and possibilities in artistic activities 28–30
 professional use of 49, 54, 278, 279–80, 284–7
 and psychological danger 234
 and team consulting 228
 and therapeutic approaches 21
 and work with clients 43, 205
rituals in counseling 55–6
Rogers, C. 40, 75, 270
Rorty, R. 272
Roscher, W. 245
Rosen, S. 256
Rubin, Alec 246

Saß, H. 106
salutogenesis 216–18
Satir, V. 256, 270
Schiepek, G. 193, 208, 210, 211, 271
Schiffer, E. 151, 217, 226
Schleiermacher, F. 20
Schlippe, A. von 181
Schnebel, D. 142
Schulte, R. 20
Schwarzbauer, M. 245
self-checking in counseling sessions 93–4
self-organization 193, 206, 208–9, 210–11, 212–13
sense activities 31–2
sensitivity raising in counseling sessions 123–8
Simon, F.B. 25
social constructivism 270–2
sociometry 248
solution-oriented approaches
  artistic activity as 40–2
  attention on success 174
  and change 42
  in counselling sessions 174, 176, 197, 198
  and crystallization principle 247
  and different expressions 44, 45–6
  and Focus on Solutions 255, 256–7
  and problem coupling 262–3
  and professional development 279–80, 281–2, 285
  resources for 42
  therapists approach to 46–7, 51
solutions of the second order 162–3
Steiner, T. 92
Stierlin, H. 181
Stige, B. 121
studio atmosphere enhancements 128–42
substitution model 214–16
supervision in decentering 221–3
surface in decentering 147–50
sustainability in decentering 201–5
Swiss Network for Solution-Oriented Work 35
synergetics 206
systems theory 193, 206, 207–8, 256–7, 269–70
Szeemann, H. 243

team consulting 226–32
theme near- and theme far-decentering 142–4
third-party artistic activities 195–6
third-party assignments 92–3
time horizons in counseling sessions 111–12
time limitations in counseling sessions 101–2
transference in counseling 79–80
transpersonal aspects of artistic activities 250–1
transitions in behavior patterns 209–10
Tschacher, W. 73, 193
Tüpker, R. 63

uncompleted assignments 176–8
unstable situations 234–5
utopian goals 116–17

Varela, F.J. 209

Watzlawick, P. 62, 205, 256
White, M. 26, 99, 182, 183, 266–8, 273
work-oriented approaches
  appreciative curiosity in 43
  and art therapies 238–9
  and artistic activities 41
  description of 45
  and Intermodal Decentering 48
  and play 190
  and work-related didactics 132–3
work-related didactics 132–8